Emergency Management in Neurology

W0050898

Series Editor
Elio Agostoni
Milano, Italy

This book series provides the reader with detailed information and guidance on the practical multidisciplinary management of the neurological patient in the emergency setting. A wide range of neurological emergencies are covered, and attention is also focused on management in specific patient groups. Numerous clinical cases are referred to in order to explain more clearly different aspects of practical management, and flow charts of the diagnostic and therapeutic approach are presented for all of the neurological conditions considered. The multidisciplinary nature of patient care is highlighted, with inclusion of a specific algorithm for each professional figure involved in the management.

More information about this series at http://www.springer.com/series/13912

Giuseppe D'Aliberti • Marco Longoni
Cristina Motto • Valentina Oppo
Valentina Perini • Luca Valvassori
Simone Vidale

Ischemic Stroke

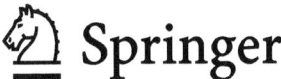 Springer

Giuseppe D'Aliberti
ASST Grande Ospedale
Metropolitano Niguarda
Milano, Italy

Marco Longoni
ASST Grande Ospedale
Metropolitano Niguarda
Milano, Italy

Cristina Motto
ASST Grande Ospedale
Metropolitano Niguarda
Milano, Italy

Valentina Oppo
ASST Grande Ospedale
Metropolitano Niguarda
Milano, Italy

Valentina Perini
ASST Grande Ospedale
Metropolitano Niguarda
Milano, Italy

Luca Valvassori
ASST Grande Ospedale
Metropolitano Niguarda
Milano, Italy

Simone Vidale
Sant'Anna Hospital
Como, Italy

ISSN 2367-1076   ISSN 2367-1084   (electronic)
Emergency Management in Neurology
ISBN 978-3-319-31704-5   ISBN 978-3-319-31705-2   (eBook)
DOI 10.1007/978-3-319-31705-2

Library of Congress Control Number: 2016957361

This Springer imprint is published by Springer Nature
The registered company is Springer International Publishing AG Switzerland

Presentation of the Series

Emergency in Neurology: A Practical Approach is a series of books which deal with the most significant chapters in the scenario of neurological emergencies, in terms of diagnosis, differential diagnosis and therapy. One particularity of the philosophy of all the books is the close integration between the strictly clinical-scientific aspects and the organizational elements, which are so important for the efficiency and effectiveness of the treatment.

The main themes of the individual volumes are as follows:

- Ischemic stroke
- Hemorrhagic stroke
- Acute loss of consciousness
- Emergencies in neuromuscular diseases
- Neurological emergency during pregnancy
- Neurological emergency in paediatrics
- Delirium, stupor and coma
- Neurological infections
- Spinal emergencies
- Cerebral hyper/hypotension syndrome
- Diagnostic tools in neurological emergencies
- Emergency medical network in neurological disease

All the volumes are structured in the same way, each containing the following chapters:

A. The first chapter is an overview of the most recent progress in diagnosis and therapy, including the clinical, instrumental and therapeutic aspects of the acute pathology under discussion, focusing specifically on the best clinical practices.

B. A chapter dedicated to clinical pathways and the associated organizational elements, following principles which inspired the international guidelines.
C. A review of clinical cases that are typical of the diverse clinical situations presented daily to the doctors involved in managing neurological emergencies. After the presentation of each clinical case, the reader finds a series of questions and topics regarding the case's management, and some observations by the co-ordinator of the series.
D. A section dedicated to the differentiated algorithms used for decision-making, based on the organizational, structural and technological features of the hospital receiving the clinical case. This final section of each book is extremely important for the day-to-day handling of neurological emergencies. This chapter aims to supply the reader with all the elements necessary to apply the guidelines and send the patient on the best clinical pathway, taking into consideration the diagnostic and therapeutic opportunities available.

The aim of this series is to provide the specialist with a useful tool for improving the outcome for patients with acute and/or time-dependent neurological pathologies, by choosing a dedicated clinical pathway according to the best practices and scenarios of the professional and organizational opportunities offered by the clinical centres.

Elio Agostoni, MD
Department of Neurosciences
ASST Grande Ospedale
Metropolitano Niguarda
Milano, Italy

Preface

The acute phase of ischaemic stroke is a time-dependent neurological emergency. Management of the stroke requires a complex series of programmes and timely actions which can assure that the process is efficient and the treatment effective. Since December 2014, scientific literature regarding acute stroke has been enriched with new evidence which broadens the range of treatment offered, from simple thrombolysis to a combination of the procedures of venous thrombolysis and mechanical thrombectomy. This scenario makes it ever more necessary to have a dedicated organization whose objective is to guarantee the best treatment for patients with acute stroke, always and everywhere.

This volume aims to provide the specialist with a tool of reference which will help him to send the acute stroke patient along the pathway in the most efficient and coherent manner, taking directions from scientific literature and International Guidelines. The scope of stroke management is extremely complex, and its developments are a fundamental point of reference for directing diagnostic, clinical and instrumental choices, for selecting the patients who qualify for the best therapy and for defining the aspects of their prognosis. This book applies a dynamic methodology to deal with current diagnostic aspects and the latest directions in the guidelines. Real clinical cases are introduced which record the various stages of the problems, the diagnostic-therapeutic decisions and the patients' clinical pathways: the decision to include these cases derived from observing the daily reality, which is then presented to the reader in a critical way through the reflections and comments of clinical experts.

The importance of this book lies in its determination to put the best clinical practices into real-life contexts, without losing sight of the organizational characteristics of the hospitals receiving the acute stroke victim.

In keeping with this concept, the diagnostic-therapeutic pathways for acute stroke are differentiated according to the hospitals' technical, professional and structural characteristics. The philosophy of this volume places the reader in a real situation and offers the clinical expert the chance to choose the best pathway, also considering the functional features of the hospital where the case is to be handled. This paradigm facilitates the development of pathological networks and broadens the concept of the 'Hub and Spoke' organization for accurately managing acute ischaemic stroke as a time-dependent pathology. Making up for any avoidable delay is the basic element, and it starts with a good organization which will help the patient's clinical outcome. In this scenario, the structural and organizational characteristics of the clinical centres are used to differentiate the clinical pathways for patients with acute stroke, thus facilitating the clinical expert in his choices and highlighting the importance of operative cooperation between the centres in the network.

Milan, Italy   The Series Editor and the Authors

Contents

Abbreviations

ACA	Anterior cerebral artery
ACAS	Asymptomatic Carotid Atherosclerosis Trial
ACE	Angiotensin-converting enzyme
ADC	Apparent diffusion coefficient
AHA	American Heart Association
AIFA	Italian Drug Agency
AMI	Acute myocardial infarct
aPTT	Activated partial thromboplastin time
ASA	American Stroke Association
ASPECTS	Alberta Stroke Program Early CT Score
BP	Blood pressure
CBF	Cerebral blood flow
CBG	Capillary blood glucose
CBV	Cerebral blood volume
CCO	Contralateral carotid occlusion
CEA	Carotid endarterectomy
CI	Confidence interval
CT	Computerized tomography
CVA	Cerebrovascular accident
DWI	Diffusion-weighted imaging
ECG	Electrocardiogram
EEG	Electroencephalography
EMA	European Medicines Agency
ESO	European Stroke Organization
FDA	Food and Drug Administration
GPP	Good practice point
GRE	Gradient echo
HR	Heart rate
ICA	Internal carotid artery

ICD	Intracardiac device
ICP	Intracranial pressure
INR	International normalized ratio
ISO	Italian Stroke Organization
MCA	Middle cerebral artery
MRI	Magnetic resonance imaging
mRS	modified Rankin Scale
MTT	Mean transit time
NASCET	North American Symptomatic Carotid Endarterectomy Trial
NIHSS	National Institute of Health Stroke Scale
NMR	Nuclear magnetic resonance
NNT	Number needed to treat
NOACs	New oral anticoagulants
NYHA	New York Heart Association
OAT	Oral anticoagulant therapy
OR	Odds ratio
PT	Prothrombin time
PTT	Partial thromboplastin time
PWI	Perfusion-weighted imaging
rtPA	Recombinant tissue-type plasminogen Activator
SPREAD	Stroke Prevention and Educational Awareness Diffusion
TIA	Transient ischaemic attack
TT	Thrombin time
WHO	World Health Organization

Contributors

Elio Agostoni, MD Division of Neurology and Stroke Unit, Department of Neuroscience, ASST Grande Ospedale Metropolitano Niguarda, Milano, Italy

Giuseppe D'Aliberti Department of Neuroscience, Department of Neurosurgery, ASST Grande Ospedale Metropolitano Niguarda, Milano, Italy

Marco Longoni Department of Neuroscience, Department of Neurology and Stroke Unit, ASST Grande Ospedale Metropolitano Niguarda, Milano, Italy

Cristina Motto Department of Neuroscience, Department of Neurology and Stroke Unit, ASST Grande Ospedale Metropolitano Niguarda, Milano, Italy

Valentina Oppo Department of Neuroscience, Department of Neurology and Stroke Unit, ASST Grande Ospedale Metropolitano Niguarda, Milano, Italy

Valentina Perini Department of Neuroscience, Department of Neurology and Stroke Unit, ASST Grande Ospedale Metropolitano Niguarda, Milano, Italy

Luca Valvassori Department of Neuroscience, Department of Neuroradiology, ASST Grande Ospedale Metropolitano Niguarda, Milano, Italy

Simone Vidale Division of Stroke Unit and Neurological Emergiences, Sant'Anna Hospital, Como, Italy

Chapter 1
Brief Description of Recent Developments in Diagnosis and Treatment

Simone Vidale, Giuseppe D'Aliberti, and Luca Valvassori

1.1 Introduction

World Health Organization (WHO) defines stroke as the sudden onset of neurological symptoms attributable solely to a brain disorder and caused by a circulatory disorder lasting more than 24 h.

In Western countries, stroke is the leading cause of severe disability in adults and the third cause of death [1].

At present, therefore, the scientific community is committed to actions dedicated to improving the prognosis in terms of mortality and residual disability.

1.2 Diagnosis

In order to deliver the best possible treatment, correct diagnosis is needed in the earliest stages after onset of symptoms. In this respect, at least three elements are of vital importance in the early evaluation of patients with suspected ischaemic stroke: medical history, neurological examination and neuroimaging. The first factor focuses mainly on accurately gathering data about the timing of the onset of symptoms, allowing the medical staff to synthesize the alleged timing of intracranial arterial occlusion. This

G. D'Aliberti et al., *Ischemic Stroke*, Emergency Management in Neurology, DOI 10.1007/978-3-319-31705-2_1,
© Springer International Publishing Switzerland 2017

factor is essential in order to practise the best possible therapy, as will later be explained.

1.2.1   Clinical Neurological Evaluation

The initial diagnostic classification is not possible without an objective neurological evaluation. Cerebral ischaemia in different vascular territories can present with specific clinical syndromes, some of which are already pathognomonic of the aetiology responsible for the event. Lacunar syndromes are particularly recognizable, totally or partially affecting the anterior arterial territory, and syndromes related to posterior vascular territories. In this regard, the National Institute of Health proposed in the past a rating scale (National Institute of Health Stroke Scale – NIHSS), based on the execution of an objective neurological evaluation, allowing the clinical severity of the disease at onset to be synthesized in one number (Table 1.1) [2]. The higher the value, the higher the clinical severity. Today this scale is the most universally used, and it is also standardized in different languages, so that it can be applied in different countries. In addition, the value of the NIHSS is also a criterion for the administration of thrombolytic therapy. Since, as previously mentioned, stroke is the leading cause of disability in adults, to date the modified Rankin Scale (mRS, Table 1.2) has been taken into account to exemplify this condition through a numerical value (Table 1.1). Conventionally, grades 0–1 express total independence, but many trials consider a value on the mRS of between 0 and 2 (box) as a favourable outcome [3].

1.2.2   Neuroradiological Diagnosis

In the acute phase of stroke, the instrumental techniques of neuroimaging are intended to exclude pathologies like stroke (stroke mimics) and to distinguish ischaemic lesions from haemorrhagic lesions, to assess the volume of damaged brain

TABLE 1.1 National Institute of Health Stroke Scale (NIHSS) and modified Rankin Scale (mRS)

NIH Stroke Scale

1a	Level of consciousness	0	Alert
		1	Not alert; but arousable by minor stimulation
		2	Not alert; requires repeated stimulation
		3	Responds only with reflex motor or autonomic effects or totally unresponsive
2a	LOC questions	0	Answers both correctly
		1	Answers one question correctly
		2	Answers neither question correctly
1c	LOC commands	0	Performs both tasks correctly
		1	Performs one task correctly
		2	Performs neither task correctly
2	Best gaze	0	Normal
		1	Partial gaze palsy
		2	Forced deviation
3	Visual	0	No visual loss
		1	Partial hemianopia
		2	Complete hemianopia
		3	Bilateral hemianopia
4	Facial palsy	0	Normal
		1	Minor paralysis
		2	Partial paralysis (near- or total paralysis low face)
		3	Complete paralysis of one or both sides

TABLE 1.1 (continued)

NIH Stroke Scale			
5	Motor arm	0	No drift
	(a) Left arm	1	Drift
	(b) Right arm	2	Some effort against gravity
		3	No effort against gravity
		4	No movement
		UN	Amputation
6	Motor leg	0	No drift
	(a) Left leg	1	Drift
	(b) Right leg	2	Some effort against gravity
		3	No effort against gravity
		4	No movement
		UN	Amputation
7	Limb ataxia	0	Absent
		1	Present in one limb
		2	Present in two limbs
		UN	Amputation
8	Sensory	0	Normal
		1	Mild-to-moderate sensory loss
		2	Severe-to-total sensory loss
9	Best language	0	No aphasia
		1	Mild-to-moderate aphasia
		2	Severe aphasia
		3	Mute, global aphasia

(continued)

TABLE 1.1 (continued)

NIH Stroke Scale

10	Dysarthria	0	Normal
		1	Nil-to-moderate dysarthria
		2	Severe dysarthria
		UN	Intubated
11	Extinction and inattention	0	No abnormality
		1	Visual, tactile, auditory, spatial, personal inattention
		2	Profound hemi-inattention or extinction in more than one modality

From: http://www.NINDS.nih.gov

TABLE 1.2 Modified Rankin Scale

Description	Score
No symptoms at all	0
No significant disability despite symptoms	1
Slight disability	2
Moderate disability	3
Moderately severe disability; unable to walk without assistance	4
Severe disability; bedridden, incontinent and requiring constant nursing care and attention	5
Dead	6

parenchyma and, finally, to identify the vascular lesion responsible for neurological deficit. The development of technology in the field of neuroradiology has allowed the use of advanced computerized axial tomography (CAT) and nuclear magnetic resonance (NMR), which distinguish the irreversibly damaged brain parenchyma from that which is potentially recoverable through rapid recovery of its vasculature. Although these methods have a theoretically significant impact also on the choice of therapy, such surveys are strongly dependent on their availability in some centres, and their effective role in therapeutic decision-making is still under investigation.

Computerized Tomography (CT)

Basal CT Scan

The CT scan is certainly the most widespread method of radiological investigation, and its advantages are primarily attributable to the speedy acquisition of images. In the hyperacute phase of stroke, the CT brain scan without contrast is the prime investigative method for excluding stroke mimics and haemorrhagic lesions, which would obviously lead to a completely different management of the patient. With this objective, the CT brain scan has proven highly sensitive. Furthermore, prompt execution of the CT scan on all patients with suspected stroke has proved to be the strategy with the best cost-effectiveness ratio in the management of these patients. The sensitivity of this investigation increases after the first 24 h from onset of symptoms. However, some previous studies showed a 61 % prevalence of early signs of cerebral ischaemia on CT [4]. The main early signs are shown in Fig. 1.1. The presence of these factors is significantly associated with worse prognosis (odds ratio [OR], 3.11; 95 % confidence interval [CI], 2.77–3.49). In particular, middle cerebral artery (MCA) hyperdense signs, which indicate the presence of a thrombus within the lumen of the arterial vessel, can be observed in approximately 30 % of ischaemic stroke patients in the territory of the same artery [5]. Although, as mentioned above, these early signs are associated with a worse clinical outcome, it is currently not completely clear how these factors should be considered when deciding whether or not to administer intravenous thrombolytic therapy [6]. Experienced

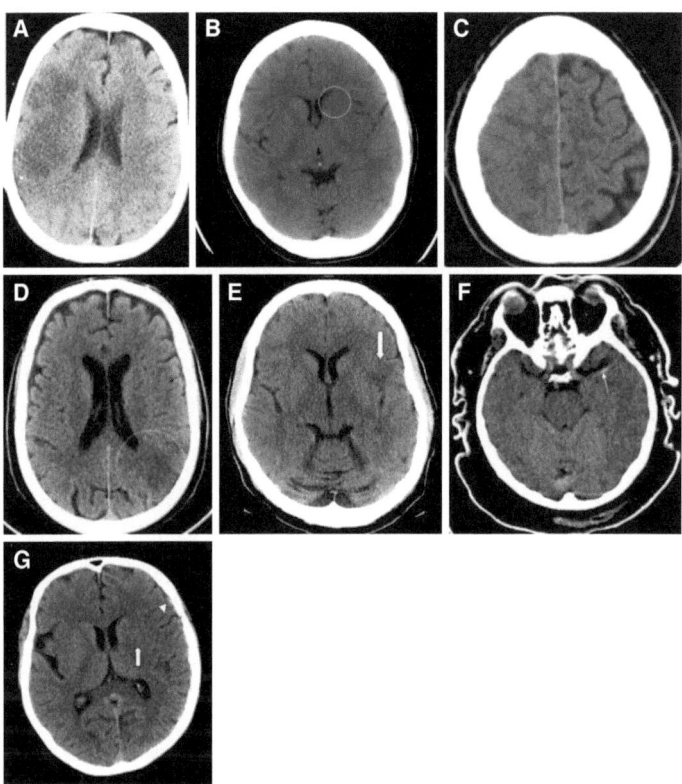

FIGURE 1.1 Early signs on brain CT scan without contrast medium: (**a**) more than 1/3 cerebral parenchymal hypodensity in the medial cerebral artery territory. (**b**) Lenticular nucleus hypodensity. (**c**) Cortical sulcal effacement. (**d**) Focal parenchymal hypodensity. (**e**) Loss of the grey-white matter difference in the basal ganglia region. (**f**) Hyperdensity of large vessels (e.g. hyperdensity of cerebral media). (**g**) Loss of the insular ribbon or obscuration of the Sylvian fissure

radiologists, neuroradiologists and neurologists can recognize these signs, although previous studies showed some difficulties in identifying them [7]. Standardized methods such as the Alberta Stroke Program Early CT Score (ASPECTS) have been developed in order to recognize early ischaemia [8].

TABLE 1.3 Assignment ASPECTS score

The middle cerebral artery is divided into ten regions
The subcortical structures have a score of 3, each divided into caudate, lentiform nucleus and internal capsule
The cortex pertaining to the middle cerebral artery has a score of 7: 4 points deriving from the axial cut at basal ganglia level for insular cortex, region M1, region M2 and region M3 and 3 points deriving from the next cut with each one for regions M4, M5 and M6
One point is subtracted for each area with signs of early ischaemia (hypodensity or oedema)
A normal brain CT scan has a score of 10, while widespread ischaemia corresponds to ASPECTS 0

ASPECTS has been developed to provide a simple and reproducible method for identifying early ischaemic changes at parenchymal level, which have been identified on CT scan. The value of this scale is derived from the evaluation of two axial cuts on the CT scan: one at the level of the thalamus and basal nuclei, and the other at the level of the rostral basal nuclei. The methodology for calculating the ASPECTS scale score is presented in Table 1.3.

Although the use of the ASPECTS score helps in selecting patients, above all for endovascular treatment in the acute phase, it does not apply to the lacunar score, to ischaemia in the midbrain or to other ischaemic lesions involving arterial territories other than the MCA.

The advent of next-generation or multi-slice CT scans has increased the speed at which images are acquired and also means that intra- and extracranial arteries can be evaluated on a CT angiography. Furthermore, spiral CT scan is a technology that allows integration of conventional image acquisition with functional elements, such as perfusion methods; early assessment of the canalization level of the arteries and of parenchymal perfusion can be checked immediately after a basal CT scan and over a period of 5–10 min [9].

CT Angiography

This method is used to observe and verify that the main extra- and intracranial arterial branches are correctly canalized. After rapid intravenous administration of a bolus of contrast medium, the CT scan acquires the images of how the contrast medium is distributed in the cranial vascular district and high-lights any filling defects of the artery corresponding to the presence of a thrombus occluding the same vessel. This instrumental method currently is a highly important management element for the potential administration of therapy in the acute phase of an ischaemic stroke and in particular for choosing to carry out mechanical thrombectomy. Study of the cerebral pial collateral circulation can be performed through the use of a multiphase CT angiography that allows the images to be acquired in three different phases after administering the contrast medium: (1) acquisition of images from the aortic arch to the summit during arterial peak, (2) acquisition during the intermediate venous phase and (3) acquisition during the delayed venous phase [10]. Unlike the perfusion CT scan (see below), multiphase CT angiography means the whole brain can be included, reducing any possible background 'noise' created by the patient moving and allowing rapid assessment of collateral circulation, and, finally, there is no need for any further contrast medium. In a recent trial, multiphase CT angiography was used in order to positively select the patients to be given mechanical thrombectomy (ESCAPE trial) [11]. In addition to these purposes, this kind of method allows the patency of the extracranial carotid system to be studied while simultaneously looking for any stenosis or obstructions that may justify the acute event observed.

CT Perfusion

The volume of the entire brain perfusion can be mapped through intravenous administration of a bolus of contrast medium. With this method, scanning is repeated over time in the same portion of the cerebral parenchyma, according to where the bolus of contrast medium passes through the arterial wall [12]. The images displayed need to be analysed and interpreted. Hypodense areas correlate to cerebral ischaemic regions. In addition, quantitative analysis of the kinetics of the contrast medium through the brain allows estimation of the cerebral blood flow (CBF), cerebral blood volume (CBV) and mean transit time (MTT) necessary for the blood to pass from the vascular compartment through the cerebral tissue [13]. The limit values of CBF and CBV might be used to predict whether the brain parenchyma will be able to survive or if they will die; however, there are no validated and standardized limit values at the moment. Applying the ASPECTS method to CBF or MTT mapping seems to identify the maximum extension of ischaemia in absence of reperfusion, and the difference between CBV and CBF (or MTT) on the ASPECTS scale seems to identify the area of ischaemic penumbra, that is, the brain tissue that can potentially be saved [10].

Nuclear Magnetic Resonance

Unlike the CT scan, basal magnetic resonance imaging (MRI) needs more time to acquire and reconstruct images. For this reason, it is difficult to use in an emergency-urgency situation, and therefore it cannot be included in the protocol of acute stroke patient management. However, this radiological method has 100 % diagnostic accuracy in detecting haemorrhagic lesions [14], and some particular sequences such as gradient echo (GRE) can distinguish acute alterations from chronic forms. Protocols that combine T1 and T2 sequences with diffusion-weighted imaging (DWI), perfusion-weighted imaging (PWI) and GRE can identify ischaemia even in an ultra-acute phase. This differs from the previously mentioned capacity of the CT scan.

DWI and PWI

The diffusion-weighted imaging technique is based on the capacity of the MRI to detect a signal from the movement of water molecules interposed between two close pulses of radiofrequency. This type of investigation can detect anomalies related to cerebral ischaemia within 3–30 min from onset of symptoms, when a traditional MRI and CT scan would not reveal them [15]. Any restrictions in the distinction between cytotoxic and vasogenic oedema, above all in T2 sequences of DWI, are resolved by using the apparent diffusion coefficient (ADC). ADC can quantify the extent of water diffusion. In this context, a hypointense signal in the ADC mappings corresponds to a cytotoxic oedema, while a hyperintense signal represents a vasogenic oedema. A systematic review of the literature published in 2010 concluded that the DWI method is superior to basal CT scan in the diagnosis of ischaemic stroke in patients presenting within 12 h of symptom onset [16]. The study also provided an indication of the predictive value of the clinical and functional outcomes. Since DWI shows ischaemic damage and not the ischaemia itself, PWI can identify the ischaemic area through fast NMR in order to measure the quantity of contrast that reaches the brain tissue. CBF, CBV and MTT maps are processed through several scan phases of the same area of brain parenchyma. Although the aforementioned American systematic review highlighted the association between the volume of the lesion detected by PWI and clinical severity, no evidence has emerged of the usefulness of this technique in daily use for diagnosing ischaemic stroke. Both methods, however, are of critical importance in detecting ischaemic penumbra. Accurate identification of reversible ischaemic brain damage is the key factor in selecting patients for reperfusion, with the aim of achieving the best results in terms of efficacy and safety. The classical 'mismatch' pattern between DWI and PWI highlights the cerebral parenchyma area that can still be saved. In particular, while DWI detects the irreversibly damaged brain parenchyma (ischaemic core), PWI can highlight the hypoperfused area which, subtracted from the previous one, defines the ischaemic penumbra area. Although these findings in the past were highlighted in consensus guidelines, their precise role in the management of acute stroke has not yet been clearly defined [17]. However, these laboratory investigations have some useful aspects, as described below:

1. Abnormal volumes in DWI and PWI during acute stroke correlate to initial clinical severity and final volume of the lesion [18]

2. Severe perfusion defects in mismatch areas on DWI/PWI may be a risk factor for enlargement of the lesion [19]
3. Patients with arterial occlusion disease are at higher risk of lesion enlargement through increased infarction within areas of perfusion deficit [20]
4. The significant correction of cerebral parenchymal hypoperfusion after administering fibrinolytic drugs may predict a positive outcome at 90 days from the event [21]

NMR Angiography

Similarly to CT angiography, this technique allows extra- and intracranial vessels to be visualized, highlighting any stenosis or occlusion. The percentages of sensitivity and specificity in detecting arterial steno-occlusive lesions vary widely from 86 to 97 % for CT angiography and from 62 to 91 % for MRI angiography [22]. An acute thrombolytic occlusion is usually displayed as a hypointensive image in the large vessels (middle or carotid cerebral artery).

Neurosonology

Carotid colour Doppler and transcranial Doppler are two noninvasive methods used for neurovascular assessment of big extra- and intracranial arterial vessels. In spite of the fact that they can be used rapidly and at the patient's bedside, they are rarely included in the diagnostic routine of the acute phase, where other methods such as CT angiography are favoured. The aim of assessing supra-aortic trunks (carotids and vertebral) is to underline potentially dangerous situations represented by serious stenosis or to identify the cause of stroke, such as, for example, occlusion of a vessel or arterial dissection. A transcranial Doppler visualizes Willis intracranial circulation. This diagnostic instrument is based on the emission of low frequency-pulsed sounds that penetrate through bone windows. This method allows the identification of stenosis, occlusions, collateral circuits and possible reperfusion after a thrombolytic treatment. There are some limitations that lead to this method rarely being applied in urgency. Among these limitations are the experience of the operator, problems in finding the bone window and low potentiality on posterior circulation. Because of these reasons, CT angiography is preferred in clinical practice in urgency, as it is extremely rapid and accurate.

Conventional Angiography

Traditional angiography is rarely used in the acute phase of stroke, unless there is a clear indication for endovascular treatment for reperfusion; this technique is to date the principal and most accurate technique for studying extra- and intracranial circulation. In fact, it can detect stenosis; occlusions; dissections; inflammatory conditions, such as vasculitis; etc. [22]. With cerebral angiography, we can study collateral circulations and the degree of cerebral perfusion. In emergencies, the use of cerebral angiography is limited in particular because of the availability of some valid alternatives, such as CT angiography, which can supply a vascular picture that is sufficiently accurate to help make the necessary therapeutic decisions. However, cerebral angiography has a higher level of sensitivity and diagnostic specificity than other less invasive methods, especially for occlusions of large arterial vessels. However, through angiography, it is possible to combine pharmacological and mechanical endovascular therapeutic reperfusion procedures.

1.3 Therapy

The main objective of acute stroke treatment is to save as much of the cerebral parenchyma as possible in order to minimize residual disability in the medium and long term after the acute event. Therefore, the main goals of treatment in the acute phase of ischaemic stroke concern two main aspects: (1) The attempt to bring the situation of arterial occlusion back to its previous condition of vessel patency, improving the supply of oxygen and glucose correlated to artery reperfusion; (2) To block dysmetabolic processes which, in an anaerobic environment, contribute to the increase in volume of the infarction of brain parenchyma. In the acute phase of stroke, vascular reperfusion and neuroprotection treatments should be practised respecting the concept of maximum urgency of intervention. The scenario of the therapy offered also includes more invasive procedures requiring surgery. Very briefly, these interventions (e.g. carotid thromboendarterectomy) are aimed at reducing the risk of early recurrence of stroke and preventing deterioration of the anatomical and clinical situation. Another range of surgical procedures (decompressive craniectomy, placement of external ventricular deviation) aim at preventing clinical deterioration in the presence of intracranial hypertension due to the 'mass' effect of the lesion.

1.3.1   Reperfusion Treatment

Early recanalization of occluded arteries with thrombolytic therapy is the most efficient procedure for protecting the brain parenchyma which is not yet infarcted. While lysis of the thrombus occluding the vessel is the immediate result that is pursued through this procedure, improvement in terms of clinical outcome is the final objective of such treatment. An earlier meta-analysis published in 2002, which analysed the data of 2006 patients, confirmed the positive predictive role of recanalization in achieving a positive outcome after 3 months (OR, 4.43; 95 % CI, 3.32–5.91), as well as in reducing death (OR, 0.24; 95 % CI, 0.16–0.35) [23]. In the same meta-analysis, 24.1 % of the patients showed spontaneous recanalization. However, the highest percentages of reperfusion were observed in the group of patients treated with mechanical thrombectomy (83.6 %), followed by a combination of systemic and locoregional therapies (67.5 %) and the intra-arterial procedure (63.2 %). Several factors are associated with favourable recanalization. First of all, size and location of the thrombus: higher volumes of thrombus, or thrombosis of the large vessels of previous atherosclerotic stenosis, seem to be factors for resistance to thrombolysis, as well as involvement of the extracranial internal carotid, occlusions in the carotid artery or the T basilar artery [13, 24–27]. The status of pial collateral circulation is also a factor that affects the success of reperfusion of the artery. Thrombolytic treatment can be delivered in a well-defined time window, beyond which its effectiveness is significantly reduced at the expenses of safety. Patient management in the hyperacute phase of stroke must provide a quick pathway leading to prompt treatment [28]. In addition to drug therapy, recent findings have meant that therapeutic potentials can be increased by giving a positive presentation of using different devices to offer mechanical recanalization techniques to selected patients.

Endovenous Thrombolysis

Intravenous administration of alteplase (recombinant tissue-type plasminogen activator – rtPA) has proven effective in reducing disability at 90 and 180 days after stroke. However, the benefit of the drug tends to decrease significantly as time goes by, and the time window currently applied is 4.5 h. At first, alteplase was administered within 3 h from onset of symptoms because of evidence in previous studies such as NINDS, in which 38 % of the treated patients reached a favourable outcome compared to 21 % of the placebo group, with no significant increase in the risk of mortality [29]. ECASS III assessed the efficacy of the treatment by extending the time window to 4.5 h [30]. The main result of the study was the effectiveness of alteplase compared to placebo (OR, 1.34; 95 % CI, 1.02–1.76; number needed to treat [NNT], 14), with no significant difference between the two groups regarding mortality and symptomatic haemorrhages. Further evidence emerged from the SITS-ISTR observational study that confirmed data already presented in a previous randomized trial [31]. To date, no evidence has emerged from literature concerning the efficacy and safety of rtPA between 4.5 and 6 h. IST-3 is the most important trial that has taken this therapeutic window into consideration and has enrolled more than 3,000 patients [32]. It has shown that there is no temporally positive trend for a favourable outcome, and in particular, the subanalysis of 1,007 patients treated within 4.5 and 6 h has shown a statistically significant difference between the groups of treated and untreated patients (47 % versus 43 %; OR, 1.31; 95 % CI, 0.89–1.93). A previous meta-analysis published in 2012 involved over 7,000 patients treated within 6 h [33]. Globally, the results showed that thrombolytic treatment was superior to placebo (OR, 1.17; 95 % CI, 1.06–1.29), with a net benefit for those who were treated within 3 h. In fact, the patients treated between 3 and 6 h did not benefit significantly from the treatment (OR, 1–07; 95 % CI, 0.96–1.20). In conclusion, a recent meta-analysis has taken into consideration the trials previously published and has analysed the outcomes of almost 7,000 patients [34]. The main observations emerging from this analysis concern the clear benefit of receiving thrombolytic therapy within 3 h (OR, 1.75; 95 % CI, 1.35–2.27). The benefit is maintained between 3 and 4.5 h (OR, 1.26; 95 % CI, 1.05–1.51), whereas it decreases between 4.5 and 6 h (OR, 1.15; 95 % CI, 0.95–1.40). An important finding shows that the observed benefit does not depend on the patient's age or clinical severity. Taking into consideration the data mentioned above, the most relevant message for a clinician can be summarized in one general concept: early intervention in the therapeutic window is the determining factor for the effectiveness of systemic thrombolytic treatment [35, 36].

Endovascular Treatment of Stroke (Thrombolysis, Thrombectomy, Thromboaspiration)

Although intra-arterial rtPA treatment has always shown promising potential benefits in terms of clinical outcome, its effectiveness remains unproven. The positive aspects of this procedure include the possibility of administering a lower dose of drug than with systemic thrombolysis, direct visualization of vessel recanalization and above all the possibility for the patient to be treated where there are contraindications to intravenous administration of thrombolytic drugs. PROACT II was the first study carried out on a large patient population to give positive results [37]. In 2010, a meta-analysis that assessed trials comparing intra-arterial thrombolysis with other treatments (including endovenous heparin) on a total of 395 patients showed a clear benefit to clinical outcomes (OR, 2.1), even in the presence of an increase in symptomatic brain haemorrhages (OR, 2.9) [38]. More recent studies, such as the Italian randomized study 'SYNTHESIS Expansion' that compared endovenous rtPA and intra-arterial rtPA have confirmed that pharmacological endovascular treatment is no more effective than endovenous treatment (OR, 0.71; 95 % CI, 0.44–1.14) [39]. The combined thrombolytic treatment (endovenous and intra-arterial), known also as bridging therapy, is based on two positive factors which are valid for both treatments: on the one hand, speedy administration of endovenous therapy is widely available; on the other hand, intra-arterial treatment is highly effective in obtaining vessel recanalization and, consequently, a better clinical outcome. Although the theory involves the potential added value of intra-arterial therapy, the IMS III study did not find this combined approach beneficial if compared to intravenous treatment [40]. A drastic change in the treatment of acute stroke has occurred recently, with the intravascular use of mechanical devices producing a marked improvement in the patients' clinical outcome. In fact, in early 2015, the results of a series of trials which have some common characteristics were published: (1) The combined approach, endovascular and systemic; (2) The use of mechanical thrombectomy (also referred to as *stentrievers*); (3) Careful and rigorous selection of the patients based on the integration of radiological investigations aimed at identifying the site of the occlusion; (4) A well-defined time limit (which varies in the different trials) within which it is possible to administer endovenous rtPA and perform the endovascular procedure of mechanical thrombectomy. The above-mentioned trials resulted in the updated indications and recommendations for treating acute ischaemic stroke: for patients with ischaemic stroke in the territory of the anterior circulation and documented occlusion of a major vessel, intra-arterial mechanical thrombectomy is recommended by means of a stentriever device [41]. This treatment can be preceded or not by a standard treatment with intravenous rtPA. In particular, the following criteria seem to be of critical importance for this procedure:

1. Basic neuroimaging must exclude bleeding and must identify at most a small ischaemic lesion
2. Radiological examinations with contrast medium must demonstrate the proximal occlusion of a major vessel of anterior circulation
3. The therapeutic procedure must be carried out in centres with proven experience, above all in using stentriever devices
4. Mechanical thrombectomy (Table 1.4) must be performed as early as possible and potentially within 6 h from onset of symptoms

Below is the description of the most important trials that evaluated the efficacy of additional treatment with mechanical thrombectomy by means of stentriever. The MR CLEAN study included 500 patients with evidence of an arterial proximal occlusion of the anterior circulation, who were chosen at random for mechanical thrombectomy within 6 h from the onset of symptoms, versus standard treatment [42]. Approximately 90 % of the patients included in the study had previously received intravenous thrombolytic therapy. The final results have demonstrated the superiority of mechanical thrombectomy compared to standard treatment, when the clinical outcome is assessed 3 months after the event (OR, 1.67; 95 % CI, 1.21–2.30), with a NNT of 7.4. There were no significant increases in mortality rates or in symptomatic haemorrhages in the group of patients submitted to mechanical thrombectomy when compared with standard care. The ESCAPE study enrolled 316 patients with occlusion of a major artery of the anterior circulation and possibility of execution of mechanical thrombectomy up to 12 h from onset of symptoms [13]. This trial also recognized the same randomization of arms. However, the patients with a big ischaemic core on their CT scan, and those with ineffective collateral circulation were excluded. The follow-up results after 3 months showed the superiority of mechanical thrombectomy (OR, 2.6; 95 % CI, 1.7–3.8) with NNT of 4.2. The SWIFT PRIME study enrolled 196 patients aged between 18 and 80 years with ischaemic stroke caused by the occlusion of a large vessel of anterior circulation, established through radiological examination [43]. All patients were treated with endovenous rtPA within 4.5 h from onset of symptoms. Randomization provided possible mechanical thrombectomy through the Solitaire FR device. After 3 months, thrombectomy achieved a positive outcome in 60 % of the patients, versus 35 % in the control group, with NNT of 4. The EXTEND-IA trial included 70 patients [44]. Excluded from randomization were patients with an ischaemic core of over 70 ml or with no brain parenchyma which could potentially be saved. Two groups were created for randomization: one with standard treatment only and the other one with mechanic

TABLE 1.4 Main results of trials on mechanical thrombectomy

Study	Centres (*n.*)	Patients IA	EV	Good outcomes (%) IA	EV	p
MR CLEAN	16	233	267	76 (32.6)	51 (19.1)	<.01
ESCAPE	22	165	150	87 (53)	43 (29.3)	<.01
EXTEND-IA	14	35	35	25 (71.4)	14 (40)	<.01
SWIFT PRIME	39	98	97	59 (60.2)	33 (35.3)	<.01
REVASCAT	4	103	103	45 (43.7)	29 (28.2)	<.01

thrombectomy by means of Solitaire FR. Also in this case, 3 months after the event, the patients treated with mechanical thrombectomy benefitted from a more favourable outcome (71 % versus 40 %) with NNT of 3.2, with no significant difference in mortality or symptomatic brain haemorrhages. The REVASCAT study randomized 206 ischaemic stroke patients to mechanical thrombectomy within 8 h versus medical treatment only [45]. Endovascular procedure significantly reduced the rate of disability after 3 months from the event, with an improvement of the clinical outcome (44 % versus 28 % with NNT of 6.3), without significantly increasing the risk of mortality or symptomatic brain haemorrhages. On the whole, previous studies provide evidence that an early mechanical thrombectomy procedure with stentriever devices, in addition to intravenous thrombolytic treatment, is effective in reducing disability in patients with stroke caused by large arterial vessel occlusion [46, 47]. The value of NNT needed to obtain functional independence thus varies between 3 and 7.5. Unlike previous experiences and trials, careful selection of the patients to be treated with mechanical thrombectomy, in addition to systemic thrombolysis, is a key factor in achieving maximum benefit with minimum risk [48]. In particular, a basal CT scan showing evidence of occlusion of intracranial main artery (distal carotid artery, sections M1/M2 MCA or sections A1/A2 of anterior cerebral artery) and the absence of large ischaemic infarctions are two key factors in selecting patients for mechanical thrombectomy. Even in the absence of any validation indicated by the results of randomized trials and only in the light of several clinical series, another kind of arterial recanalization procedure – direct thrombus aspiration – is rapidly spreading to many centres. This therapeutic procedure consists in intracranial navigation with special intracranial catheters, which are soft but wide lumen (newly marketed), which are brought close to the thrombus. The thrombus is then sucked manually (by creating a negative pressure in the lumen) or via external mechanical aspiration pumps connected to the catheter. According to some authors, this therapeutic procedure allows a high rate of recanalization with extreme rapidity of execution.

Bleeding Complications Associated with Thrombolytic Treatment

Cerebral bleeding complications associated with thrombolytic treatment can be divided into three categories: haemorrhagic, symptomatic and asymptomatic. Symptomatic cerebral haemorrhages means cerebral haemorrhages leading to a significant deterioration of the neurological clinical situation (at least four points of NIHSS or death). Several factors are associated with the risk of suffering from a cerebral haemorrhage after thrombolysis. In particular, the advanced age of the patient and higher clinical severity at onset are two essential elements in increasing the risk of intracranial haemorrhagic complications. The NINDS study showed a significant association between clinical severity and cerebral haemorrhages (OR, 1.8; 95 % CI, 1.2–2.9); the same trial established a higher risk of cerebral haemorrhagic complications in patients with early signs of ischaemia on their basal brain CT scan, such as oedema or mass effect (OR, 7.8; 95 % CI, 2.2–27.1) [49]. Other factors – such as heart failure, hyperglycaemia, leukoaraiosis, extension of the infarction area on DWI-MR, persistence of vessel occlusion after treatment with rtPA, kidney failure and atrial fibrillation – can increase the risk of haemorrhage associated with thrombolysis [50, 51]. Atrial fibrillation is a clinical condition that requires treatment with oral anticoagulants. Several meta-analyses of clinical studies have shown that using warfarin, albeit with nontherapeutic INR values, significantly contributes to increasing the risk of cerebral haemorrhages (OR, 2.6; 95 % CI, 1.1–5.9) [52]. An analysis of an American register with over 23,000 patients did not confirm the increased risk for patients treated with anticoagulants, although their INR was below 1.7, after adjusting the model according to age, gender, clinical severity, systolic blood pressure and glycaemia [53].

1.3.2   Neuroprotection

The main aim of neuroprotective therapy in the acute phase of ischaemic stroke is to be able to modulate the complex process that follows occlusion of the artery. As different mechanisms are implicated, many factors are involved. The complexity of the neuroprotection therapeutic approach is very complex, and there are different therapeutic approaches. In particular, some major targets are recognized for neuroprotection. First, inflammation is a complex process in which many factors that determine 'self-sufficiency' of brain damage interact and contribute to increasing the size of the infarcted area. Numerous therapeutic attempts have considered targeting adhesion molecules and cytokines [54]. A second target is represented by oxidative stress, which is a key to the whole process of postischaemic damage and is not produced by inflammation alone but also by excitotoxicity that comes from an environment with low oxygen tension. Apoptosis and autophagy are very complicated processes in which transcriptional proteins and transmission molecules have been studied for producing neuroprotective substances [55]. Although some Phase II studies have shown effective results, no Phase III trials have shown, to date, any clinical benefits deriving from treatment with neuroprotective therapies.

1.3.3   Surgical Treatment

Carotid Thromboendarterectomy in Urgency and Extra- and Intracranial Bypass

Carotid endarterectomy (CEA) is a well-defined treatment for reducing the risk of stroke in symptomatic and asymptomatic patients [56, 57]. Although both the North American Symptomatic Carotid Endarterectomy Trial (NASCET) and the Asymptomatic Carotid Atherosclerosis Trial (ACAS) have demonstrated a significant reduction in the risk of stroke for patients treated with CEA compared to patients treated with medical therapy, the benefit has not yet been clarified in the subgroup of patients excluded from these studies because of comorbidity and advanced age [58, 59].

The indication for surgery in the acute phase (within the first 4 days) or urgent phase (within the first 24 h) of stroke is primarily concerned with the prevention of early recurrence in patients undergoing medical therapy and who are candidates for revascularization [60]. The benefits are linked to the possibility of removing the cause of thromboembolism, as in the case of 'soft' or 'ulcerated' plaques, or restoring normal reperfusion of the ischaemic brain tissue from 'penumbra'. Early surgical treatment seems to reduce the risk of a recurrent stroke more than surgery deferred by 3 weeks [61]. In the NASCET study, the risk of recurrence involved in referred surgery was estimated as increasing by up to 9.5 % when compared to early surgery. The latter, however, may be burdened by the possible transformation of an ischaemic stroke into a haemorrhagic one, the possible increase of cerebral oedema or by the appearance of a hyperperfusion syndrome due to sudden recovery of normal perfusion pressure. Therefore, the effectiveness of early surgery has been called into question for neurologically unstable patients and for patients with complete occlusion of the carotid artery. An additional 16 % risk of stroke and an additional 21 % risk of death were estimated, respectively, for this subgroup of patients. If the diameter of infarcted tissue increases by more than 1 cm, the risk of permanent deterioration of neurological deficit increases by a factor of 1.7. Finally, several studies have shown that the incidence of stroke and death is significantly higher in patients with 'stroke in evolution' and in those with 'crescendo TIA' (transient ischaemic attack), respectively, 20.2 % and 11.4 % when they are submitted to early surgery. Angioplasty and stenting of the carotid were originally carried out as less invasive alternative procedures to open surgery in patients with high incidence of comorbidity. Carotid Revascularization: Endarterectomy versus Stenting Trial (CREST) – whose end point was the assessment, after 4 years, of mortality and of the risk of neurological and cardiac complications in patients with carotid stenosis who were treated with surgery versus stenting – was conclusive because of the absence of a significant difference (95 % CI, 0.81–1.51; $p = 0.51$) [62]. However, this study included symptomatic and asymptomatic patients. In conclusion, the usefulness of early surgery (emergency or urgent) seems to concern clinically stable patients, with neuroimaging showing a small infarction and a wide surrounding area of 'penumbra' due to a critical subocclusive stenosis. Another indication is the appearance of an acute neurological deficit after CEA where thrombosis of disobstructed carotid is suspected (Class IIb recommendation, level of evidence B). On the contrary, in neurologically unstable patients, in those with 'stroke in evolution' or 'crescendo TIA', the efficacy of early surgery has not yet been proven (Class IIb recommendation, level of evidence B). Specific considerations concern the risk connected to TEA procedure in relation to some factors: thrombosis of contralateral carotid artery, high carotid bifurcation, the use of shunt and patch versus direct repair [63]. The risk related to CEA in the presence of a contralateral occluded carotid artery is still debated. Data analysis in the NASCET and ACAS studies showed an increase in the stroke and death rate in patients with contralateral carotid occlusion (CCO) that were treated with CEA. Dalainas et al. observed 373 patients treated with CEA in the presence of CCO [64]. The authors did not find any significant difference in perioperative stroke or death among patients with or without CCO. A similar study with similar results was carried out by Rockman et al. [65]. Also, the use of shunt during CEA is widely debated. A recently updated meta-analysis of randomized trials found no significant difference in outcomes after CEA among surgeons who routinely shunt and those who shunt selectively. In the subset of CEAs with CCO, multiple observational studies have also found no impact of shunting on stroke or death after CEA with CCO.

However, Goodney demonstrated an increased risk of stroke or death for CEA performed in the presence of CCO, and that surgeons who shunt infrequently incur an increased risk of stroke when they do shunt [66]. In fact, contralateral occlusion of the carotid, the use of shunt and patch and high carotid bifurcation are all risk factors specific to this surgery which must be related to the time necessary for disobstruction and the absence of vascular compensation (i.e. an excluded carotid terminating in the single MCA). So a number of aspects concerning monitoring and cross-clamping, in general, remain to be defined. Several studies have suggested the value of electroencephalography (EEG) findings as an index of cerebral ischaemia arising from cross-clamping. A close correlation between EEG findings and CBF measurement has been reported, and clinical experience has demonstrated that patients who do not show EEG changes tolerate temporary carotid occlusion. In the absence of EEG changes, relatively long periods of occlusion (40–50 min) are well tolerated, at least under general anaesthesia and full heparinization. In the presence of major persistent EEG changes, cross-clamping of the internal carotid artery (ICA) does not seem to be equally tolerated. In the Collice's series, under these circumstances, the incidence of neurological deficit is a function of the duration of cross-clamping: in fact, the patients who underwent clamping occlusion for 15–30 min presented temporary postoperative deficits [67]. In conclusion, CEA, when performed by experienced practitioners in substantial volume, carries a low risk for perioperative stroke or death in most patients. Although we observed a trend towards higher perioperative mortality in patients with multiple comorbid conditions, the adverse event rates noted in patients with these risk factors still fall within the range of those reported in randomized trials and within those proposed by the American Heart Association as practice guidelines, i.e., combined stroke-death rate of 3 % in patients with asymptomatic disease and 6 % in those with symptomatic disease. In other words, only centres with a perioperative complication rate of 3 % or less should contemplate surgery. Approximately, 5–10 % of the patients with carotid TIA or with minor stroke have an occlusion originating in the carotid artery, less frequently do they have an occlusion of the distal or proximal portion of the MCA. These injuries can be bypassed by anastomosing a branch of the external carotid artery, usually the superficial temporal artery, a peripheral branch of the MCA. Such collateral was developed to improve blood supply in the distal MCA bed and to reduce the risk of stroke or the severity of stroke. However, these anastomoses between the superficial temporal and middle cerebral arteries were not beneficial in preventing stroke in patients with MCA or ICA stenosis or occlusion. A recent Carotid Occlusion Surgery Study did not show additional benefits of bypass surgery when added to medical management in patients with symptomatic atherosclerotic ICA occlusion [68]. Rare reports of improvement with early bypass surgery exist as do reports of no improvement and of haemorrhagic complications. Reports of the early use of surgical embolectomy exist. In conclusion, extracranial-intracranial bypass for the treatment of ischaemic stroke has not shown to be of benefit. Endovascular approaches appear to provide a better alternative in most situations.

Decompressive Craniectomy

Approximately 10 % of ischaemic strokes are characterized by a massive hemispheric oedema taking up space, due to the occlusion of the distal carotid or M1 segment of the MCA. These patients often present with hemiplegia, forced head and eye deviation, aphasia or a contralateral neglect syndrome [69]. Despite medical treatments such as hyperventilation, mannitol, barbiturate coma and hypothermia, mortality is estimated to be between 50 and 78 %. They experience a progressive decline in their level of consciousness typically over 48 h, ultimately succumbing as a result of transtentorial herniation within 48–96 h. Decompressive craniectomy procedures have been used to relieve increased intracranial pressure (ICP) and cerebral oedema caused by a variety of pathological events. This technique was first applied in 1905. To establish objective criteria for aggressive intervention, many investigators measured ICP, once significant clinical deterioration was apparent. In an early study, patients in whom ICP values were greater than 15 mmHg did not survive the malignant infarct [70]. In subsequent studies other authors have shown that a fatal outcome occurred in most cases when the level was greater than 30 mmHg. In addition to clinical findings, neuroimaging criteria can help to identify those patients at particular risk for a malignant infarction in the early phase of their stroke. In patients with malignant cerebrovascular accident (CVA), a large area of parenchymal hypodensity in the MCA territory often shows upon the CT scans. With progressive clinical deterioration, CT-scan demonstrated signs may also include mass effect, effacement of the basal cisterns, compression of the ventricular system, a shift in midline structures and herniation of tissue through the falx, foramen magnum or tentorium. These patients present clinically with progressive deterioration of consciousness within the first 2 days. Thereafter, symptoms of transtentorial herniation occur within 2–4 days after onset of stroke. This clinical presentation is accompanied by early CT signs of major infarct during the first 12 h after stroke; as no model of medical treatment has been proven superior to the others, treatment options may vary depending on each clinic protocol. Intracranial hypertension results in decreased pressure of cerebral perfusion and therefore decreasing blood supply throughout the cerebrum. Because of the increase in mechanical pressure and ICP, other major cerebral vessels may be compressed by the expanding tissue, against dural edges or against the skull. The result is secondary ischaemia and further expansion of the infracted area. Osteodural cranial decompression can also concern patients who, after an ischaemic stroke, develop a haemorrhage caused by medical fibrinolytic therapy or patients with extended infarction who are on anticoagulants because of previous minor strokes. Monitoring of ICP has been recommended as a guide to surgical timing [71]. A measurement of greater than 25 mmHg has been used, despite attempts at medical therapy, as an indicator for surgical intervention. Increased ICP measurements are preceded by the constellation of clinical signs and symptoms constituting the 'malignant CVA syndrome'; thus, the usefulness of ICP monitoring in these cases has been questioned. However, brain tissue shifts rather than raised ICP are probably the most likely cause of the initial decrease in consciousness. The question of the optimal time window for intervention has not yet been completely elucidated. In a recent update of a Cochrane review which included the results of three major randomized studies, Flores et al. examined the effects of decompressive surgery in patients with massive acute ischaemic stroke complicated with cerebral oedema, to judge whether decompressive surgery is effective in improving survival or survival free of severe disability [72]. In this study, outcomes were death at the end of follow-up, death or disability defined as the mRS >3 at the end of follow-up, death or severe disability defined as mRS >4 at 12 months and disability defined as mRS 4 or 5 at 12 months. The results are given using the Peto OR with 95 % CI. In conclusion, decompressive surgery reduces the risk of death and the combined outcome of death or very severe disability. It should therefore be the preferred therapy in cases where this can also be assumed to be in the best interest of the patient, given that increased survival may occur at the expense of disability. Further research is needed to establish whether this intervention is beneficial in individuals over 60 years of age. There is also a need for more information about patients' utility values for different levels of disability after stroke.

References

1. Mozaffarian D, Benjamin EJ, Go AS et al (2015) Heart disease and stroke statistics—2016 update a report from the American Heart Association. Circulation 132. doi: 10.1161/ CIR.0000000000000350.
2. Adams HP Jr, Davis PH, Leira EC et al (1999) Baseline NIH Stroke Scale score strongly predicts outcome after stroke: a report of the Trial of Org 10172 in Acute Stroke Treatment (TOAST). Neurology 53:126
3. Bonita R, Beaglehole R (1998) Modification of Rankin Scale: recovery of motor function after stroke. Stroke 19:1497

4. Wardlaw JM, Mielke O (2005) Early signs of brain infarction at CT: observer reliability and outcome after thrombolytic treatment-systematic review. Radiology 235:444

5. Leys D, Pruvo JP, Godefroy O et al (2001) Prevalence and significance of early ischemic changes on computed tomography in acute stroke. JAMA 286:2830

6. Patel SC, Levine SR, Tilley BC et al (2001) Lack of clinical significance of early ischaemic changes on computed tomography in acute stroke. JAMA 286:2830

7. Wardlaw JM, Dorman JP, Lewis SC, Sandercock PA (1999) Can stroke physicians and neuroradiologists identify signs of early cerebral infarction on CT? J Neurol Neurosurg Psychiatry 67:651

8. Barber PA, Demchuk AM, Zhang J, Buchan AM (2000) Validity and reliability of a quantitative computed tomography score in predicting outcome of hyperacute stroke before thrombolytic therapy. ASPECT Study Group Alberta Stroke Programme Eraly CT Score. Lancet 355:1670

9. Parsons MW, Pepper EM, Chan V et al (2005) Perfusion computed tomography: prediction of final infarct extent and stroke outcome. Ann Neurol 58:672

10. Menon BK, d'Esterre CD, Qazi EM et al (2015) Multiphase CT angiography: a new tool for the imaging triage of patients with acute ischemic stroke. Stroke 46:3020–3035

11. Goyal M, Demchuk AM, Menon BK et al (2015) Randomized assessment of rapid endovascular treatment of ischaemic stroke. N Engl J Med 372:1019

12. Allmendinger AM, Tang ER, Lui YW, Spektor V (2012) Imaging of stroke: part 1, perfusion CT- overview of imaging technique, interpretation pearls, and common pitfalls. AJR Am J Roentgenol 198:52

13. Lev MH (2013) Perfusion imaging of acute stroke: its role in current and future clinical practice. Radiology 266:22

14. Fiebach JB, Schellinger PD, Gass A et al (2004) Stroke magnetic resonance imaging is accurate in hyperacute intracerebral haemorrhage: a multicentre study on the validity of stroke imaging. Stroke 35:502

15. Warach S, Gaa J, Siewert B et al (1995) Acute human stroke studied by whole brain echo planar diffusion-weighted magnetic resonance imaging. Ann Neurol 37:231

16. Schellinger PD, Bryan RN, Caplan LR et al (2010) Evidenced-based guideline: the role of diffusion and perfusion MRI for the

diagnosis of acute ischemic stroke: report of the Therapeutics and Technology Assessment Subcommittee of the American Academy of Neurology. Neurology 75:177

17. Hjort N, Butcher K, Davis SM et al (2005) Magnetic resonance imaging criteria for thrombolysis in acute cerebral infarct. Stroke 36:388

18. Beaulieu C, de Crespigny A, Tong DC et al (1999) Longitudinal magnetic resonance imaging study of perfusion and diffusion in stroke: evolution of lesion volume and correlation with clinical outcome. Ann Neurol 46:568

19. Neumann-Haefelin T, Wittsack HJ, Wenserski F et al (1999) Diffusion- and perfusion-weighted MRI. The DWI/PWI mismatch region in acute stroke. Stroke 30:1591

20. Rordorf G, Koroshetz WJ, Copen WA et al (1998) Regional ischemia and ischemic injury in patients with acute middle cerebral artery stroke as defined by early diffusion-weighted and perfusion-weighted MRI. Stroke 29:939

21. Chalela JA, Kang DW, Luby M et al (2004) Early magnetic resonance imaging findings in patients receiving tissue plasminogen activator predict outcome: insights into the pathophysiology of acute stroke in the thrombolysis area. Ann Neurol 55:105

22. Latchaw RE, Alberts MJ, Lev MH et al (2009) Recommendations for imaging of acute ischemic stroke: a scientific statement from the American Heart Association. Stroke 40:3646

23. Rha JH, Saver JL (2007) The impact of recanalization on ischaemic stroke outcome: a meta-analysis. Stroke 38:967

24. Goyal M, Menon BK, Derdeyn CP (2013) Perfusion imaging in acute ischemic stroke: let us improve the science before changing clinical practice. Radiology 266:16

25. Zangerle A, Kiechl S, Spiegel M et al (2007) Recanalization after thrombolysis in stroke patients: predictors and prognostic implications. Neurology 68:39

26. Georgiadis D, Oehler J, Schwarz S et al (2004) Does acute occlusion of the carotid T invariably have a poor outcome? Neurology 63:22

27. Vidale S, Arnaboldi M (2014) Treatment of basilar artery occlusion. Ann Neurol 74:161

28. Burns JD, Green DM, Metivier K, DeFusco C (2012) Intensive care management of acute ischaemic stroke. Emerg Med Clin North Am 30:713

29. Kwiatkowski TG, Libman RB, Frankel M et al (1999) Effects of tissue plasminogen activator for acute ischaemic stroke at one year. National Institute of Neurological Disorders and Stroke Recombinant Tissue Plasminogen Activator Stroke Study Group. N Engl J Med 340:1781

30. Hacke W, Kaste M, Bluhmki E et al (2008) Thrombolysis with alteplase 3 to 4.5 hours after acute ischemic stroke. N Engl J Med 359:1317

31. Wahlgren N, Ahmed N, Dávalos A et al (2008) Thrombolysis with Alteplase 3–4.5 h after acute ischaemic stroke (SITS-ISTR): an observational study. Lancet 372:1303

32. IST-3 collaborative group, Sandercock P, Wardlaw JM et al (2012) The benefits and harms of intravenous thrombolysis with recombinant tissue plasminogen activator within 6 h of acute ischaemic stroke (the third international stroke trial [IST-3]): a randomised controlled trial. Lancet 379:2352

33. Wardlaw JM, Murray V, Berge E et al (2012) Recombinant tissue plasminogen activator for acute ischaemic stroke: an updated systematic review and meta-analysis. Lancet 379:2364

34. Emberson J, Lees KR, Lyden P et al (2014) Effect of treatment delay, age, and stroke severity on the effects of intravenous thrombolysis with Alteplase for acute ischaemic stroke: a meta-analysis of individual patient data from randomised trials. Lancet 384:1929

35. Saver JL, Fonarow GC, Smith EE et al (2013) Time to treatment with intravenous tissue plasminogen activator and outcome from acute ischaemic stroke. JAMA 309:2480

36. Vidale S, Agostoni E (2014) Thrombolysis in acute ischaemic stroke. Brain 137:e281

37. Furlan A, Higashida R, Wechsler L et al (1999) Intra-arterial prourokinase for acute ischaemic stroke. The PROACT II study: a randomized controlled trial Prolyse in Acute Cerebral Thromboembolism. JAMA 282:2003

38. Lee M, Hong KS, Saver JL (2010) Efficacy of intra-arterial fibrinolysis for acute ischemic stroke: meta-analysis of randomized controlled trials. Stroke 41:932

39. Ciccone A, Valvassori L, Nichelatti M et al (2013) Endovascular treatment for acute ischaemic stroke. N Engl J Med 368:904

40. Broderick JP, Palesch YY, Demchuk AM et al (2013) Endovascular therapy after intravenous t-PA versus t-PA alone for stroke. N Engl J Med 368:893

41. Powers WJ, Derdeyn CP, Biller J et al (2015) AHA/ASA Focused Update of the 2013 Guidelines for the Early Management of Patients With Acute Ischaemic Stroke Regarding Endovascular Treatment: a Guideline for Healthcare Professionals From the American Heart Association/American Stroke Association. Stroke 46(10):3020–3035

42. Berkhemer OA, Fransen PS, Beumer D et al (2015) A randomized trial of intra-arterial treatment for acute ischaemic stroke. N Engl J Med 372:11

43. Saver JL, Goyal M, Bonafe A et al (2015) Stent-retriever thrombectomy after intravenous t-PA vs t-PA alone in stroke. N Engl J Med 372:2285

44. Campbell BC, Mitchell PJ, Kleinig TJ et al (2015) Endovascular therapy for ischaemic stroke with perfusion-imaging selection. N Engl J Med 372:1009

45. Jovin TG, Chamorro A, Cobo E et al (2015) Thrombectomy within 8 hours after symptom onset in ischaemic stroke. N Engl J Med 372:2296

46. Prabhakaran S, Ruff I, Bernstein RA (2015) Acute stroke intervention: a systematic review. JAMA 313:1451

47. Campbell BC, Donnan GA, Lees KR et al (2015) Endovascular stent thrombectomy: the new standard of care for large vessel ischaemic stroke. Lancet Neurol 14:846

48. Hacke W (2015) Interventional thrombectomy for major stroke–a step in the right direction. N Engl J Med 372:76

49. The NINDS t-PA Stroke Study Group (1997) Intracerebral haemorrhage after intravenous t-PA therapy for ischaemic stroke. Stroke 28:2109

50. Khatri P, Wechsler LR, Broderick JP (2007) Intracranial haemorrhage associated with revascularization therapies. Stroke 38:431

51. Whiteley WN, Slot KB, Fernandes P et al (2012) Risk factors for intracranial haemorrhage in acute ischaemic stroke patients treated with recombinant tissue plasminogen activator: a systematic review and meta-analysis of 55 studies. Stroke 43:2904

52. Miedema I, Luijckx GJ, De Keyser J et al (2012) Thrombolytic therapy for ischaemic stroke in patients using warfarin: a systematic review and meta-analysis. J Neurol Neurosurg Psychiatry 83:537

53. Xian Y, Liang L, Smith EE et al (2012) Risks of intracranial hemorrhage among patients with cute ischemic stroke receiving warfarin and treated with intravenous tissue plasminogen activator. JAMA 307:2600

54. Reza Noorian A, Nogueira R, Gupta R (2011) Neuroprotection in acute ischaemic stroke. J Neurosurg Sci 55:127

55. Sahota P, Savitz SI (2011) Investigational therapies for ischaemic stroke: neuroprotection and neurorecovery. Neurotherapeutics 8:434

56. Brott TG, Halperin JL, Abbara S et al (2011) 2011 ASA/ACCF/AHA/AANN/AANS/ACR/ASNR/CNS/SAIP/SCAI/SIR/SNIS/SVM/SVS Guideline on the Management of Patients With Extracranial Carotid and Vertebral Artery Disease. Circulation 124:e54

57. Ferguson GG, Eliasziw M, Barr HW et al (1999) The North American Symptomatic Carotid Endarterectomy Trial: surgical results in 1415 patients. Stroke 30:1751

58. Executive Committee for the ASYl11ptomatic Carotid Atherosclerosis Study (1995) Endarterectomy for asymptomatic carotid artery stenosis. JAMA 273:1421

59. Huber R, Müller BT, Seitz RJ, Siebler M, Mödder U, Sandmann W (2003) Carotid surgery in acute symptomatic patients. Eur J Vasc Endovasc Surg 25:60

60. Paty PS, Darling RC 3rd, Feustel PJ et al (2004) Early carotid endarterectomy after acute stroke. J Vasc Surg 39:148

61. Brott TM, Hobson RW, Howard G et al (2010) Stenting versus endarterectomy for treatment of carotid-artery stenosis. N Engl J Med 363:11

62. Rockman C (2004) Carotid endarterectomy in patients with contralateral carotid occlusion. Semin Vasc Surg 17:224

63. Dalainas I, Nano G, Bianchi P, Casana R, Malacrida G, Tealdi DG (2007) Carotid endarterectomy in patients with contralateral carotid artery occlusion. Ann Vasc Surg 21:16–22, Med 2010;363(1):11e23

64. Rockman CB, Su W, Lamparello PJ, Adelman MA, Jacobowitz GR, Gagne PJ et al (2002) A reassessment of carotid endarterectomy in the face of contralateral carotid occlusion: surgical results in symptomatic and asymptomatic patients. J Vasc Surg 36:668

65. Bond R, Rerkasem K, Counsell C, Salinas R, Naylor R, Warlow CP et al (2002) Routine or selective carotid artery shunting for carotid endarterectomy (and different methods of monitoring in selective shunting). Cochrane Database Syst Rev CD000190

66. Goodney PP, Wallaert JB, Scali ST et al (2012) Impact of practice patterns in shunt use during carotid endarterectomy with contralateral carotid occlusion. J Vasc Surg 62:61

67. Collice M, Arena O, Fontana RA, Mola M, Galbiati N (1986) Role of EEG monitoring and cross-clamping duration in carotid endarterectomy. J Neurosurg 65:815
68. Grubb RL Jr, Powers WJ, Clarke WL et al (2013) Surgical results of the Carotid Occlusion Surgery Study. J Neurosurg 118:25
69. Ropper AH, Shafran B (1984) Brain edema after stroke: clinical syndrome and intracranial pressure. Arch Neurol 41:26
70. Schwab S, Aschoff A, Spranger M et al (1996) The value of ICP monitoring in acute hemispheric stroke. Neurology 47:393
71. Poca MA, Benejam B, Sahuquillo J et al (2010) Monitoring intracranial pressure in patients with malignant middle cerebral artery infarction: is it useful? J Neurosurg 112:648
72. Flores SC, Berge E, Whittle IR (2012) Surgical decompression for cerebral edema in acute ischaemic stroke Cochrane Database Syst Rev 1:CD003435. doi:10.1002/14651858.CD003435

Chapter 2
Clinical Cases

Marco Longoni, Giuseppe D'Aliberti, Valentina Oppo, and Luca Valvassori

In this chapter, a series of clinical cases explanatory of the various conditions relating to the pathology are collected and presented.

2.1 Case Study No. 1

Presentation of the case of a 62-year-old male. Medical history: hypertension, dyslipidaemia and smoking. He was being treated with aspirin, angiotensin-converting enzyme (ACE) inhibitor and statin. The patient presented to the emergency department of a high-complexity hospital (Hub) with global aphasia and mild paresis of the right-side limbs. These symptoms appeared after a long car voyage and during physical exertion. The neurological disorders started at 20:45; the call to the emergency services was made at 20.50. The prehospital transportation was assigned the maximum severity code, called the "stroke code", which means that the receiving hospital is put on pre-alert. The patient arrived at the emergency department at 21.25, and the neurologist was already present to receive him. At admission, the patient was alert and collaborating; global aphasia could be observed, along with eye deviation to the left, and central deficit of the VII cranial nerve. NIHSS = 9/42: 0-2-1-0-0-1-(0-0-0-0)-0-0-3-2-0. A blood sample was taken for urgent tests and a 12-lead ECG was carried out. Blood pressure was 130/80; heart rate was 70 and rhythmic, and oxygen saturation 97 % in ambient air. At 21.45, the patient was given a brain CT scan without

G. D'Aliberti et al., *Ischemic Stroke*, Emergency Management in Neurology, DOI 10.1007/978-3-319-31705-2_2,
© Springer International Publishing Switzerland 2017

contrast and a CT angiography with triphasic technique in order to study the collateral circulations.

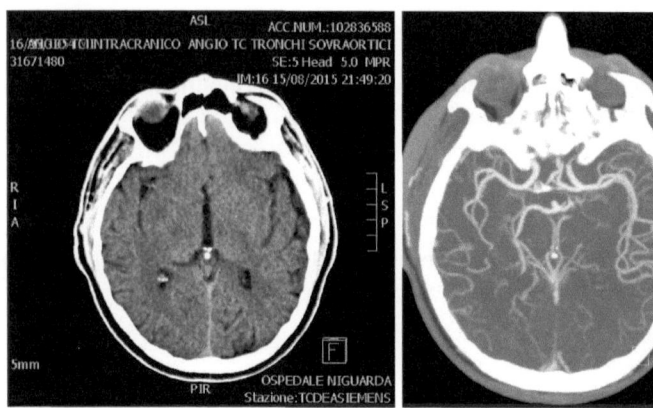

Alberta Stroke Program Early Computed Tomography (ASPECT) score 10. CT angiography shows no occlusion of large extra- and intracranial arteries.

After discussing the case, it was agreed that there were no indications for endovascular treatment with mechanical thrombectomy. At 22.00, systemic thrombolytic therapy was begun (Actilyse 76.5 mg, of which 7 mg in endovenous bolus and 69.5 mg in continuous endovenous infusion for 60 min). In the meantime, the results of the blood tests arrived, which were normal. Clinical evolution during administration of Actilyse, measured with National Institut of Health Stroke Scale (NIHSS), was as follows:

At 22.15: HT(Hyper tension) 130/80; NIHSS = 7/42
At 22.30: HT 140/80; NIHSS = 7/42
At 22.45: HT 120/80; NIHSS = 7/42
At 23.00: HT 130/75; NIHSS = 7/42

While Actilyse was being given, there was continuous monitoring of blood pressure, heart rate and oxygen saturation. Blood pressure was measured every 5 min and a clinical neurological evaluation was made every 15 min. At the end of systemic thrombolytic therapy, the patient was transferred to the stroke unit. 24 h after onset of symptoms, the brain CT scan without contrast was checked.

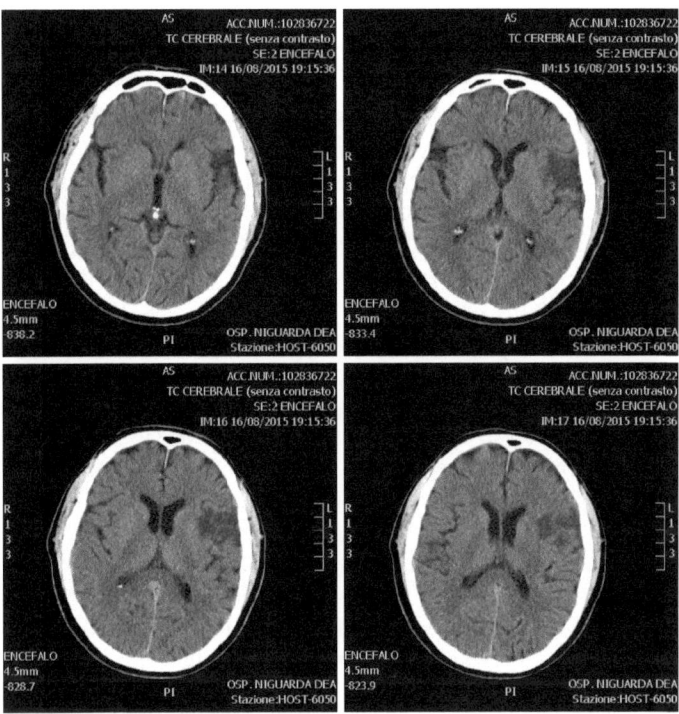

Hypodense area in the partial territory of the left middle cerebral artery.

Antiplatelet therapy was started with 100 mg/day of aspirin. After 24 h, the NIHSS was 4/42. From a clinical viewpoint, the patient was alert, could pronounce some words and could understand and follow simple orders. There was complete remission of the hemiparesis of the right side. The clinical evolution after 7 days was favourable, with further improvement of NIHSS = 2/42.

2.1.1   Topics of Discussion

- How useful is the "stroke code" in the pre- and in-hospital pathway of the patient with acute stroke?

   The "stroke code", meaning the code for maximum severity for both the pre- and in-hospital pathway, is the most important variable for reducing times in the entire pathway and for minimizing the problem of avoidable delay, as a fundamental organizational moment for the clinical outcome of the acute stroke patient [1]. In various clinical studies, applying the "stroke code", to both prehospital transportation and in-hospital pathway [2], makes it more likely that stroke patients in the acute phase will be offered the best therapy. In other words: the "stroke code" is a system variable which is absolutely indispensible for a good clinical outcome [3–5].

• What is the role of triphasic CT angiography in diagnosing stroke in the acute phase?

CT angiography is a speedy method which identifies the location and extension of the arterial occlusion. The use of CT angiography is decisive in choosing the best revascularization therapy (systemic thrombolysis versus a combined therapy of venous thrombolysis and mechanical thrombectomy). Furthermore, studying vascular anatomy via CT angiography allows the medical staff to plan the strategy for endovascular treatment. Last, but not least important, is that the use of the triphasic technique (extra-intracranial arterial phase, venous phase and late intracranial phase) can reliably establish the presence of collateral circulations. The recent ESCAPE trial (see Chap. 1) on mechanical thrombectomy versus medical therapy used this method in patient selection, demonstrating how the presence of collateral circulations is related to a good outcome and means that the therapeutic window can be extended.

2.2   Case Study No. 2

Presentation of the case of a 51-year-old male. Medical history: hypertension, metabolic syndrome and smoking (40 cigarettes per day), under therapy with ACE inhibitor. At 05.30 in the morning, the patient arrived independently at the emergency department of a high-complexity hospital (Hub) because of onset of stroke, which occurred at 04.00 with left hemisyndrome deficit. The neurologist evaluated the patient at 05.40 and at 05.43 contacted the neurovascular interventionist. The objective neurological exam found loss of visual stimulus of the left hemifield, deficit of the VII left cranial nerve, hemiplegia of the left arm and paresis of the left arm. NIHSS=11/42=0-0-0-0-0-2-(0-4-0-2)-1-0-1-1=11. At 06.05, the patient was given a brain CT scan without contrast and a CT angiography with triphasic technique.

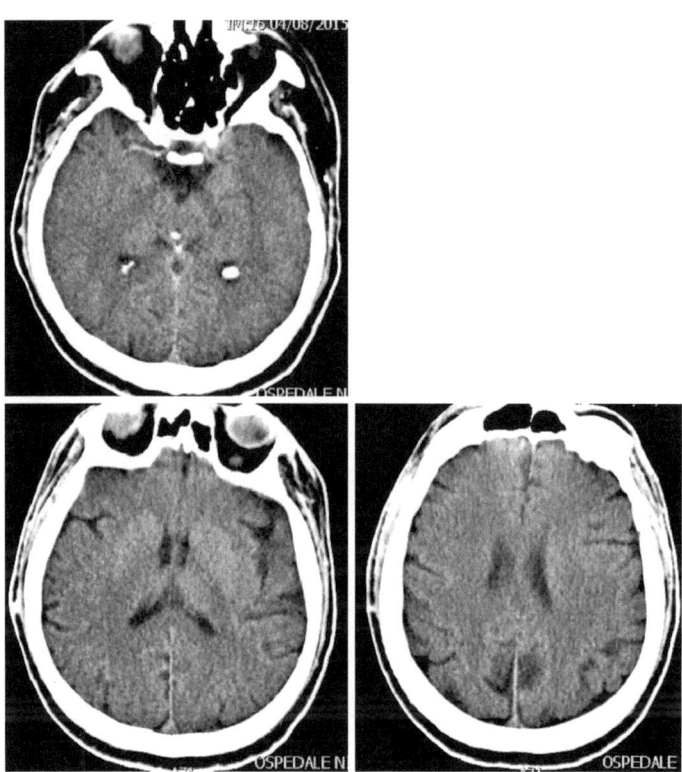

ASPECT 9/10 (hypodensity of the right-side basal nuclei), hyperdensity of the right-side MCA.

CT angiography: occlusion of the internal right carotid artery at origin (not shown in the image) caused by a coarse atheromatous fibro-calcified plaque. The intracranial extremity of the carotid is revascularized by the ophthalmic artery, with evidence of occlusion in the M1 segment of the right middle cerebral artery and good compensatory circulations via the usual anastomoses.

At 06.20, blood pressure was 140/85, NIHSS=11/42. Systemic thrombolytic therapy was begun with 81 mg of Actilyse, of which 8 mg in bolus and 73 mg in continuous endovenous infusion for 60 min. At the same time, preparations were made to transport the patient to the angiograph room. Clinical evolution during administration of Actilyse was as follows:

At 06:35: NIHSS = 11/42
At 06:50: NIHSS = 11/42
At 07:05: NIHSS = 11/42

The patient arrived in the angiograph room at 07.20. The first series of angiographic images were carried out at 07.41.

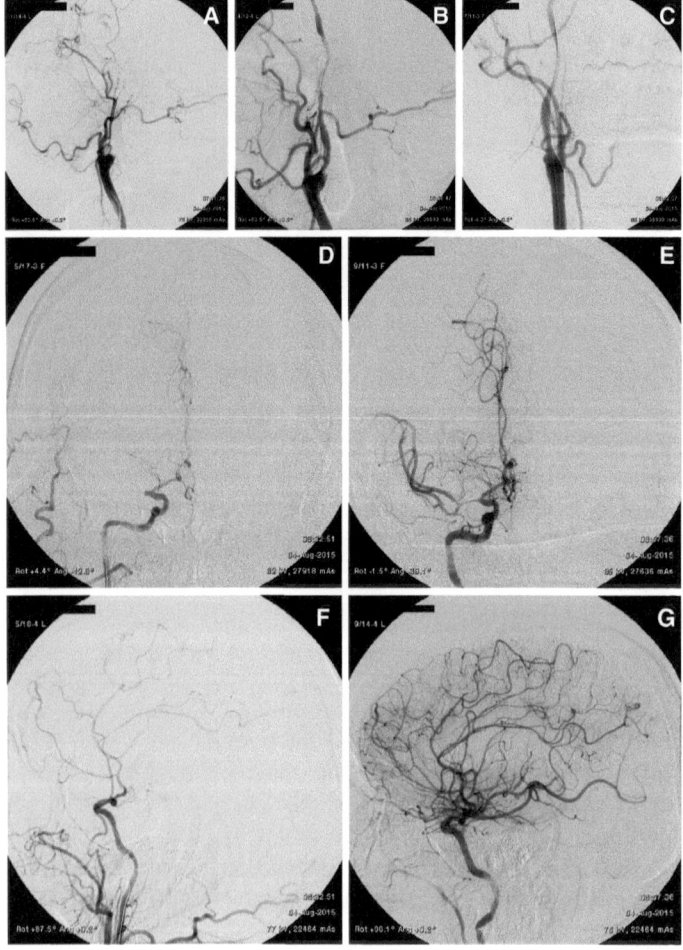

Description of the procedure: the preliminary angiograph confirmed an occlusion of the internal right carotid artery at origin (Image a) and embolic occlusion of segment M1 of the homolateral middle cerebral artery (Images d–f). A micro guide was then passed through the occluded vessel, various dilations were carried out with an angioplasty balloon and a stent was released to guarantee the vessel's patency (Images a–c). A thrombus aspiration catheter was then inserted as far as the middle cerebral artery, behind the thrombus, which was then removed via aspiration thus completely reopening the hemispheric circulation (Images e–g).

The procedure was concluded at 09.10. NIHSS = 2/42 at the end of the procedure. There remained a trace of central-type deficit of the VII left cranial nerve and a modest loss of strength in the left arm.

A post-angiography brain CT was carried out, which showed no haemorrhagic complications. A bolus of abciximab 22.5 mg (0.25 mg/kg) was then administered and a 12-h continuous infusion of endovenous abciximab (dose 0.125 ug/kg/min diluted in 50 ml of saline solution). Twenty-four hours later, double antiplatelet therapy was introduced using aspirin and ticlopidine. The patient was given an NMR.

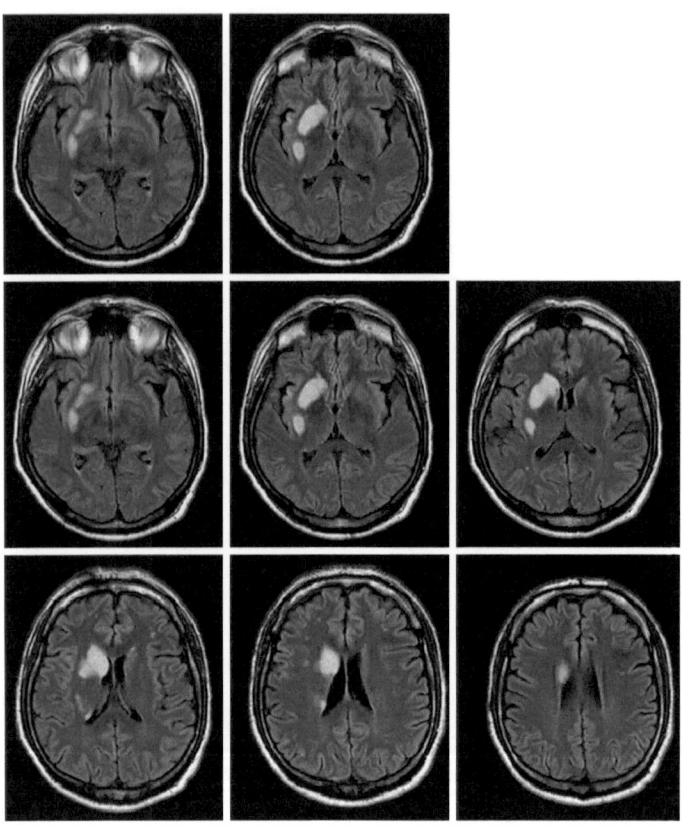

The NMR showed only an ischaemic lesion concerning the lentiform nucleus and the right periventricular region.

Clinical evolution after 5 days was decidedly favourable (NIHSS = 0, mRS = 0, BI 100).

2.2.1   Topics of Discussion

- How successful is endovenous thrombolysis likely to be, taking into consideration the morphological data of the CT angiography?

Taking into account the evidence that venous throm-bolysis is not very effective in cases of tandem occlusion (as in the present clinical case), the setting of the angiogra-phy room must immediately bc activated, and endovenous fibrinolysis should in any case be initiated.

- Is the use of a carotid stent appropriate in the acute phase?

There is very limited evidence supporting treatment of the acute phase with angioplasty and stenting of the extra-cranial segment of the carotid: that is, a few retrospective series of cases which do however show that this procedure is effective and relatively safe in selected cases [6, 7]. Although, we must not overlook the fact that insertion of a stent means that antiplatelet therapy must be started immediately [8, 9].

- Would it be appropriate to use antiplatelets less than 24 h after thrombolysis?

Using antiplatelets in the first 24 h after acute stroke is controversial [10]; in fact, not only has no benefit ever been demonstrated, but there is evidence to associate this practice with increased mortality, as well as with haemor-rhagic phenomena (see Chap. 4 and the ARTIS study). In the case we are referring to, antiplatelet therapy was administered in consideration of the elevated risk of thrombosis of the stent in a patient who, from a clinical point of view, presented a deficit which had improved almost totally (NIHSS = 2).

2.3   Case Study No. 3

Presentation of the case of a 62-year-old man. Medical his-tory: smoking, hypertension and known bilateral carotid ste-nosis. The patient arrived at the emergency department because of recurrent TIA in the right carotid arterial terri-tory. The neurological examination at the emergency department was normal. The ABCD risk assessment score = 2. The patient was given a CT scan without contrast in urgency.

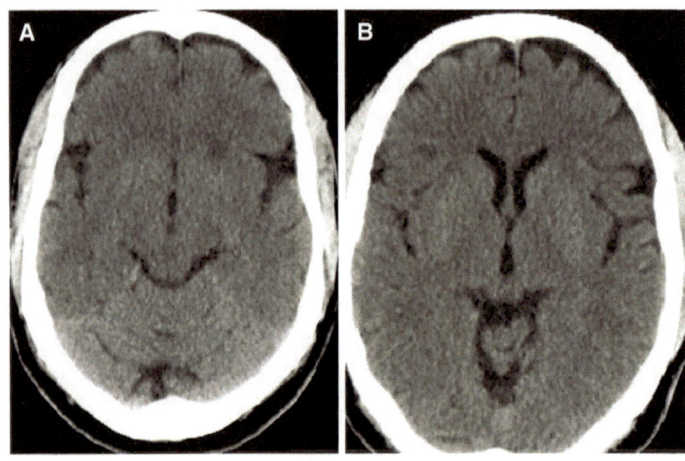

ASPECT Score 10/10.

An extracranial arterial Doppler was performed at the patient's bed. It highlighted a right carotid bulb stenosis, with a significant acceleration of flow velocity up to 240 cm/s, corresponding to a >70 % stenosis. The patient was submitted to CT angiography.

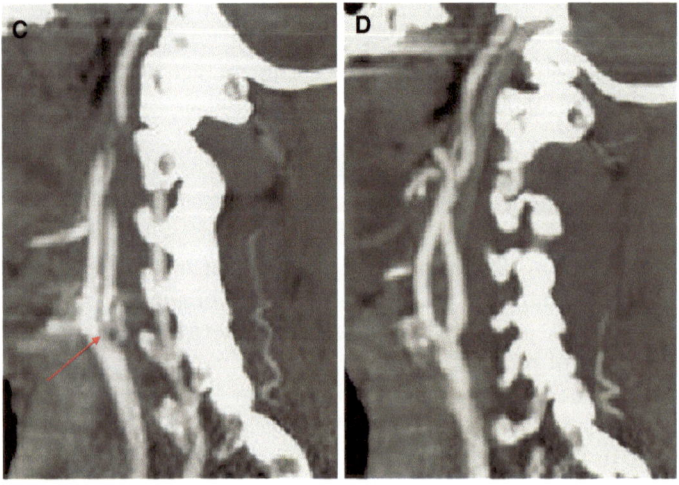

Atheromatous plaque of the right carotid bulb with reduction of the vessel lumen of 70 % (Fig. C, arrow), in addition to a nonsignificant stenosis of the left carotid bulb (Fig. D).

On the basis of this evidence, the patient was proposed for early surgery with treatment of carotid thromboendoarterectomy on the third day. The patient underwent preoperative cerebral angiography.

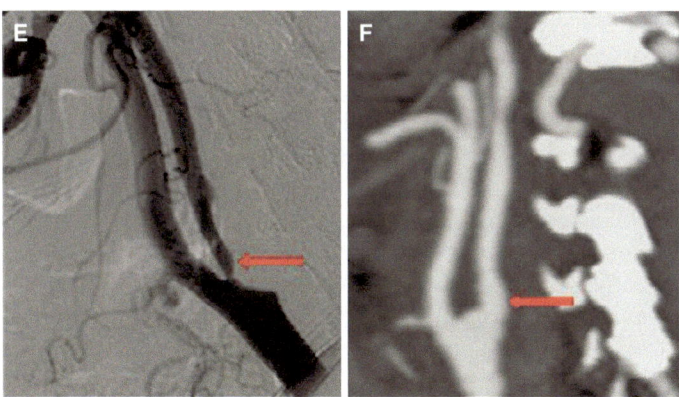

Figure E shows the stenosis on preoperative angiography, on the right.

Figure F shows the post-operatory result.

The patient had a regular postoperative recovery and was discharged on the fifth day.

2.3.1   Discussion

- Timing of carotid surgery in urgency.
  Although not supported by evidence level I, we think that carotid surgery should be performed as early as possible. The selection criteria for the patient to be submitted to carotid revascularization have already been described in Chap. 1, to which reference is made.
- What instrumental investigations are necessary in patients undergoing carotid surgery?

Patients with indication for carotid surgery must undergo carotid Doppler study in addition to an instrumental method of neuroimaging (CT angiography or MRI angiography). Angiography is performed only in selected cases when there is a discrepancy between the two methods or clinical indecision persists.

2.4   Case Study No. 4

Presentation of the case of a 64-year-old man. Medical history: ischaemic cardiopathy in dilated-hypokinetic evolution (New York Heart Association [NYHA] III).

The patient suffered from diabetes, had carried a ventricular assistant device (HeartMate II) since 2009 and was a candidate for a heart transplant (Status 2A). Blood group B positive. The patient carried an intracardiac device (ICD). He was suffering from polidistrectual vasculopathy and had a history of tubulovillous adenoma of the colon which had been removed endoscopically in 2012. He was under therapy with the following drugs: ACE inhibitor, beta-blocker, Cardio Aspirin, dipyridamole, omeprazole, folic acid, statins and warfarin. The patient arrived at the emergency department because of a sudden fall at 23.15 caused by the sudden onset of left hemiplegia. He was transported to the emergency department via EMS with a red code assigned to the transportation. The patient arrived at the emergency department at 00.36. At 00.48, he was given a brain CT scan without contrast.

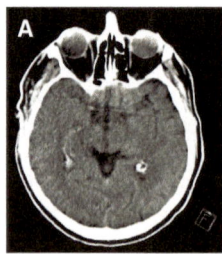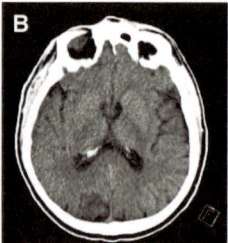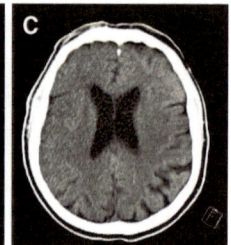

ASPECT 10/10 (Fig. A–C).

At 1.10, the neurological clinical assessment of the patient highlighted the following information: the patient was vigilant, oriented in time and space. Furthermore, he showed dysarthria, right head deviation, left hemiplegia with hemi-hypoaesthesia, Babinski on the left and extinction at double visual and tactile stimulus (NIHSS = 16/42 (0,0,0,2,0,2,4,0,4, 0,0,1,0,1,2). At 1.20, a triphasic CT angiography was performed.

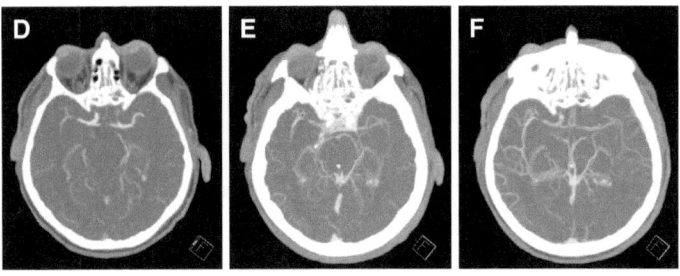

CT angiography result: right middle cerebral artery occlusion in the pre-bifurcation section (Fig. D, E) with good collateral circulation visible in the intermediate phase (Fig. F).

At 1.40, the patient was transferred to the angiography room.

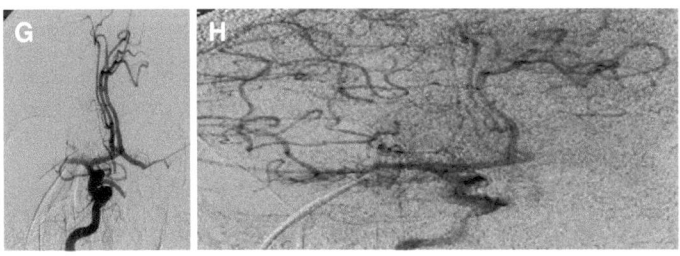

At 3.10, the first angiographic series confirmed the occlusion of the right middle cerebral artery with good collateral circulation through leptomeningeal collateral vessels (Fig. G, H).

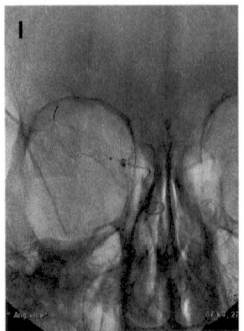

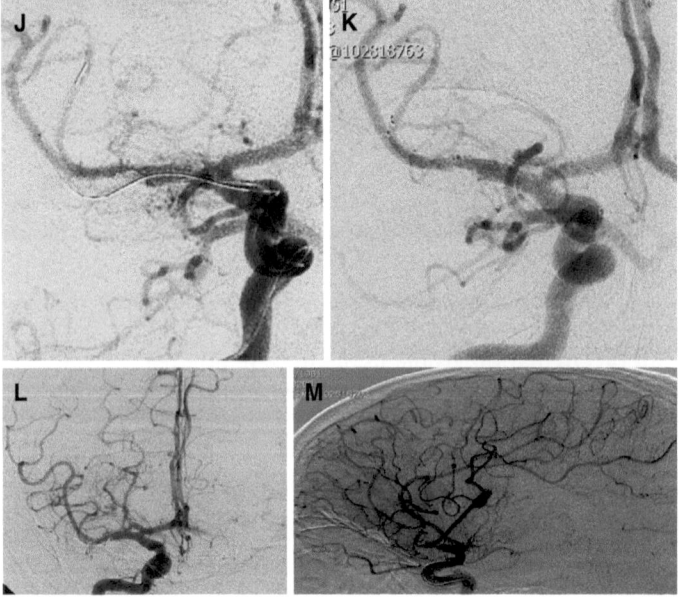

Thromboaspiration and removal of the blood clot were carried out with stent retriever (Fig. I–L). It was agreed to release an intracranial stent on the upper bifurcation branch (Fig. M). The last angiographic series at 4.40 showed patency of M1 segment of middle cerebral artery and good vascularization of the superior branch frontal destination. The patient was treated with double antiplatelet therapy and low molecular weight heparin at anticoagulant dosage.

A further post-procedure brain CT scan without contrast showed no haemorrhagic complications. The neurological examination in the stroke unit highlighted an initial improvement of motor impairment; the patient could move his upper limb in the absence of gravity and could lift his lower limb from the plane of his bed. There was an improvement in the clinical sign ocular deviation. NIHSS = 11/42 (0,0,0,1,0,2,3,0,2,0,0,1,0,1,1). On the third day, a brain CT scan without contrast was performed.

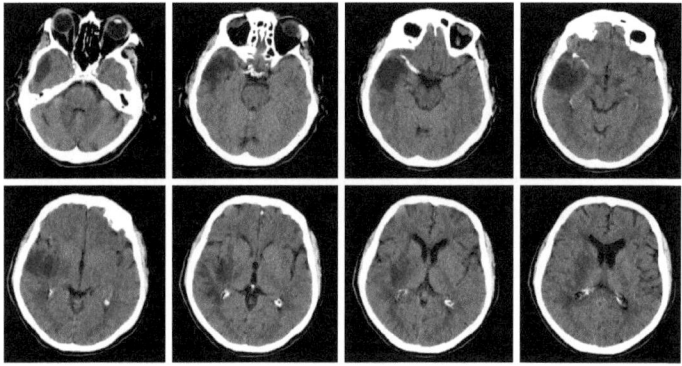

Ischaemic lesion in temporal and nucleocapsular areas.

The patient was discharged; prescribed an oral anticoagulant therapy, aspirin and dipyridamole; and sent to a rehabilitation centre. At discharge, mRS = 4. Approximately 1 month later, the patient arrived at the emergency department because of an ictal episode of aphasia and left ocular deviation. Time of onset of symptoms: h. 13.00. Time of arrival at the emergency department: h. 14.10. At 14.40, he was submitted to brain CT scan without contrast. The CT scan did not show any changes compared with the CT scan performed on admission; in particular, there was no evidence of haemorrhagic infarction. The clinical neurological examination was performed at 15.00: the patient had open eyes, was not contactable showed left gaze deviation, flexed the left upper limb, recognized pain stimulus to the right upper limb and was paraplegic.

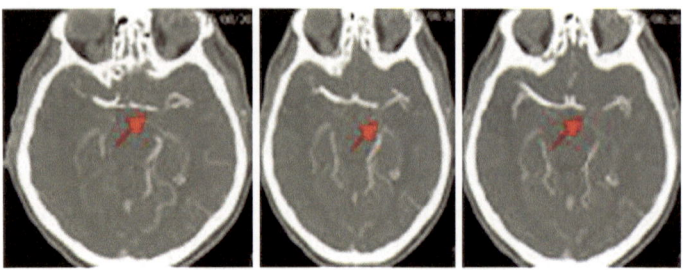

CT angiography result: the previously placed stent was patent, while the M1 segment of left middle cerebral artery was not visible (see red arrow).

In view of both the clinical conditions of the patient (mRS > 3), and the timing of the first event (minor stroke in the last 3 months), it was decided not to perform mechanical thrombectomy.

2.4.1   Discussion

- Is the decision of not re-intervening on the base of the pre-stroke disability correct?

  The limited data available in the literature is referred to systemic thrombolysis. In patients with mRS 1, 2 or >3 before the index event, there is no evidence of increase in the risk of haemorrhage after administering rtPA. On the contrary, both the probability of a good clinical outcome and the mortality rate after 3 months are higher in this group compared to patients without premorbid impairments [11].

2.5   Case Study No. 5

Presentation of the case of a 39-year-old male. Medical history: depression syndrome, migraine with aura. He was being treated with citalopram 10 mg/day. The patient presented to the emergency department of a high-complexity hospital (Hub) at 8.15. The transportation was assigned the "stroke code". The patient arrived with right side hemianopsia, motor aphasia and right side hemianopsia. Symptoms presented upon awakening at 7.15. NIHSS = 16/42: 0-2-0-0-2-2-(0-4-0-3)-0-1-2-0-0. The emergency department carried out urgent blood tests and electrocardiography with 12 derivations. A cannula was positioned into the right limb in order to perform a brain CT scan without contrast, a CT angiography and a CT perfusion (ore 8.43).

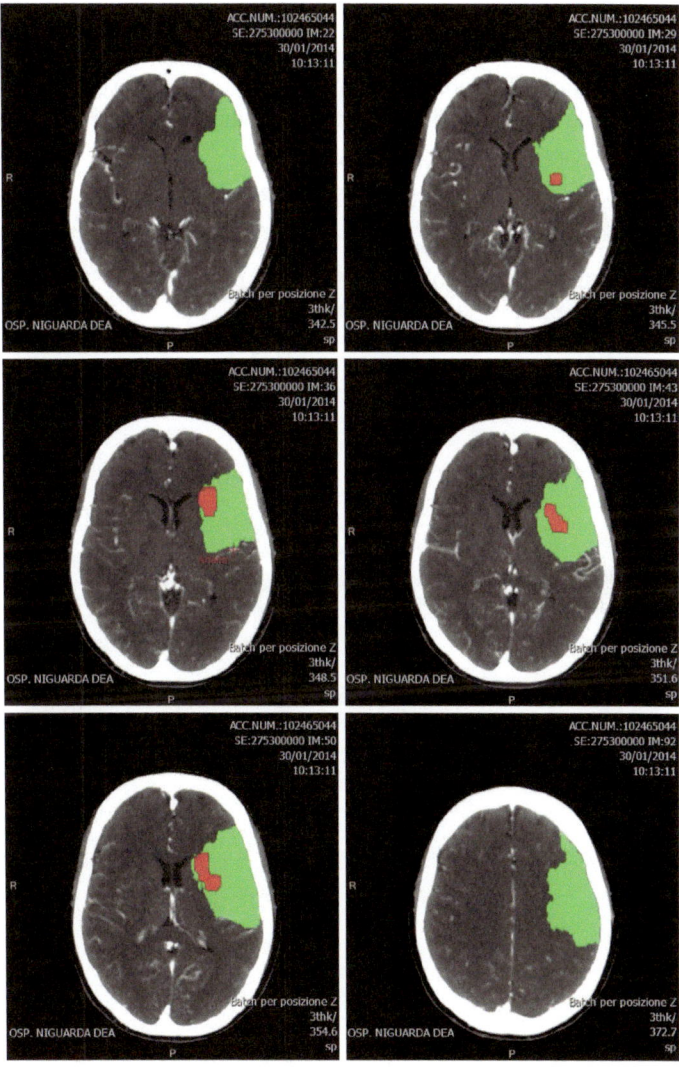

ASPECT score 10/10.

The CT angiography showed: occlusion of the upper division branch of the left middle cerebral artery. Perfusion CT scan showed: advantageous mismatch between ischaemic core and penumbra.

Since there were no absolute contraindications to intravenous thrombolysis, the patient was treated with intravenous rtPA at 9.30. The patient was administered 63 mg of Actilyse, 6 mg of which in bolus and 57 mg via continuous intravenous infusion over 60 min. Simultaneously, the patient was sent to the angiography room. During administration of Actilyse, the following clinical evolution was observed:

At 9.45: NIHSS = 16/42; BP 140/85
At 10.00: NIHSS = 16/42; BP 135/80

At 10.10, the patient was in the angiography room and intravenous thrombolysis was still in progress. At 10.35, the first angiography series was carried out.

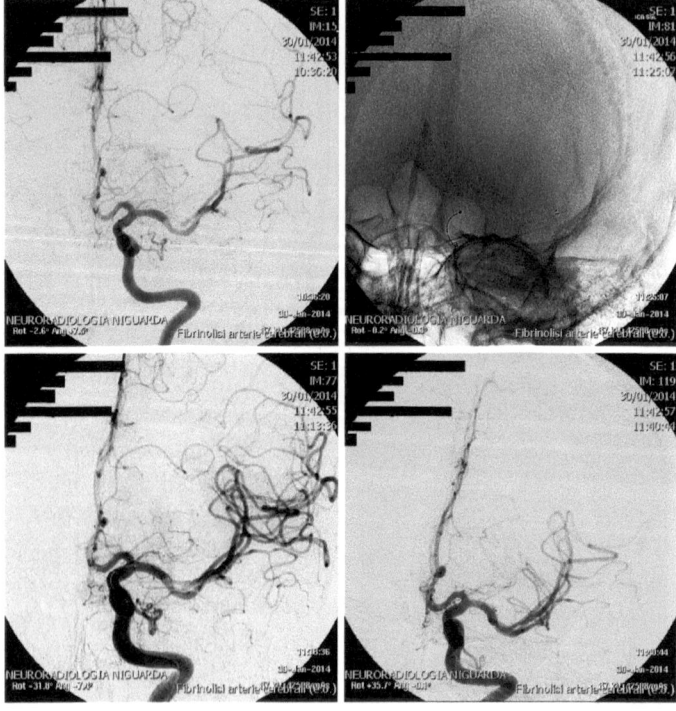

The study of the left carotid artery showed the presence of a blood clot involving the final segment M1 of the middle cerebral artery and causing the occlusion of a large branch of the upper division and the subocclusion of a third branch.

It was decided to bring a microcatheter beyond the thrombus; it was opened with a stent retriever through which the thrombus occluding the vessel was removed. In this way, the hemispheric circulation was reopened. At 11.40, the procedure ended. The patient had an immediate clinical improvement, recovering strength and speech impairment. NIHSS = 5/42: 0-2-0-0-0-1-(0-1-0-0)-0-0-1-0-0. The patient was given a brain CT scan 24 h later.

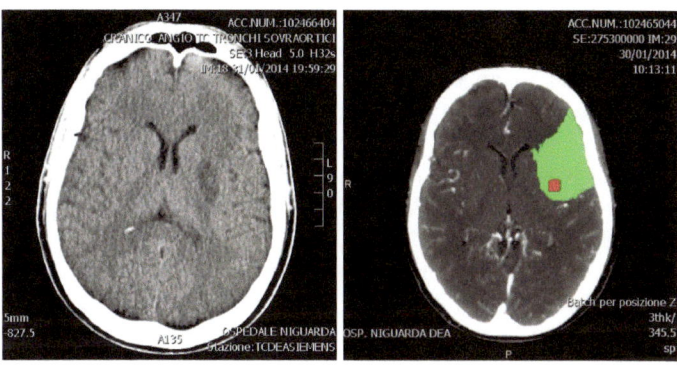

The CT scan highlighted a small deep left ischaemia, corresponding to the ischaemic core shown on the perfusion CT scan before the treatment.

The patient had a favourable clinical evolution and was discharged with NIHSS = 2/42: 0,0,0,0,0,1,(0,0,0,0),0,0,0,1,0. mRS = 2. BI = 100/100.

2.5.1   Topics of Discussion

• What is the relationship between stroke upon awakening and new imaging techniques?

  Perfusion CT scan, MRI with DWI and PWI and the study of collateral circulation by means of triphasic CT angiography are imaging techniques that can potentially highlight the ischaemic tissue that can be saved independently from the time of onset of symptoms. Such methods, as discussed in Chaps. 1 and 3, are currently not mentioned in the management of the patient in the therapeutic window, but can be useful in case of a stroke in which the time of onset of symptoms is unknown.

2.6   Case Study No. 6

Presentation of the case of a 61-year-old male. Medical history: chronic atrial fibrillation, ablation of a breast nodule in 2005 and 2006, multiple previous attempts at electrical cardioversion to no benefit, former smoker, hypercholesterolemia under medical treatment, hypothyroidism in replacement therapy and recent episode of transitory ischaemia. The patient was receiving pharmacological therapy at home, with dabigatran 150 mg×2/day, digoxin 0.25×2/day, metoprolol and simvastatin 10 ml.

The patient presented to the emergency department of a high-complexity hospital (Hub) at 07.30 in the morning, due to a suspected ischaemic left-side stroke, with neurological symptoms appearing on awakening at 07.00. In the emergency department, a neurological evaluation found the following data: the patient was alert, global aphasia was observed, with lateral right-side homonymous hemianopsia and facial-brachial paresis of the right side. NIHSS 16/42: 0-2-2-0-2-2-(0-4-0-0)-0-1-3-0-0. The patient was given a brain CT scan without contrast and a CT angiography.

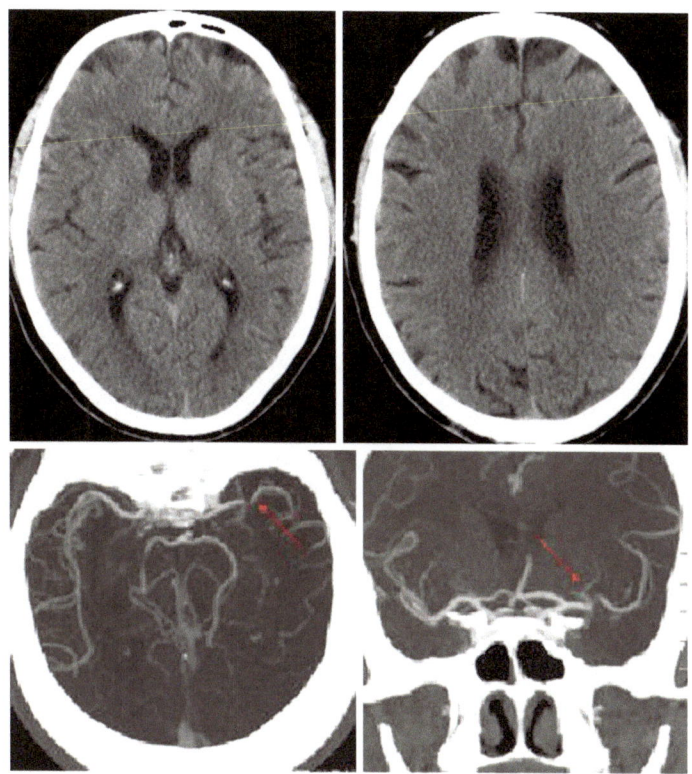

ASPECT 10/10.

The CT angiography shows subocclusive stenosis of the upper branch of the left middle cerebral artery.

Taking into consideration the therapy with new oral anti-coagulants (NOACs), as well as the fact that the time of symptom onset was unknown, the patient was excluded from endovenous fibrinolytic therapy, and no indication was found for fibrinolytic treatment. Therapy was started with antiplatelets and statin in the emergency department, and transfer to the stroke unit was organized. Tests for coagula-tion international normalized ratio (INR) and activated partial thromboplastin time (aPTT) were normal. Kits for Hemoclot or for ecarin clotting times were not available in the hospital. Clinical deterioration was observed during the second day, with impaired consciousness and loss of strength which also affected the right leg. NIHSS = 25/42: 2-2-2-0-2-2-(0-4-0-4)-0-2-3-2-0. An urgent brain CT scan was carried out.

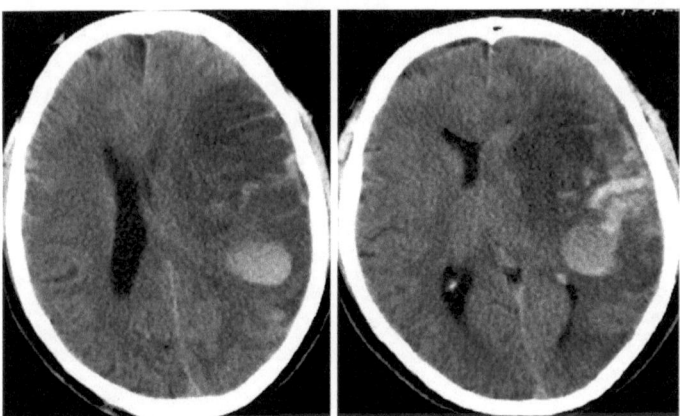

Extensive haemorrhagic infarction with midline shift and possible transtentorial uncal herniation.

The case was discussed with the neurosurgeon, and a decision was made to proceed with decompressive hemicraniectomy. A left frontal temporoparietal craniotomy was therefore begun. The dura mater was tense. On opening up the dura, a haemorrhagic and prevalently temporal infarction was evident, which was treated with surgical toilet, and good cerebral decompression was achieved. Dural synthesis was then carried out with Neuro-Patch. The operculum bone was removed to allow decompression.

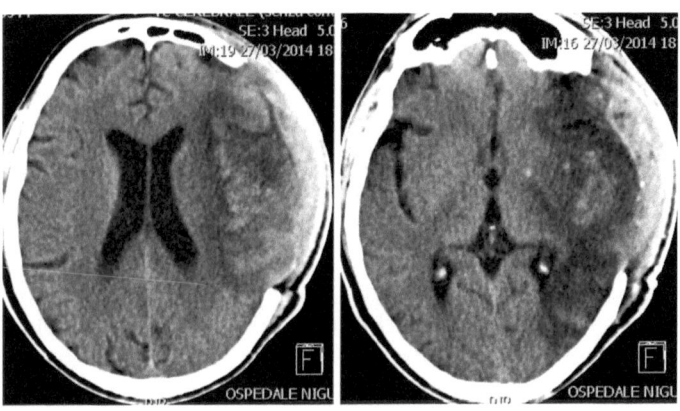

The patient was transferred to intensive therapy and his intracranial pressure monitored. While he was in neurointensive care, repeated electroencephalograms were carried out, which revealed continuous left frontal paroxysmal activity. An antiepilepsy therapy was prescribed with phenytoin and phenobarbital after an initial but ineffective therapeutic attempt using levetiracetam. The antiepilepsy therapy was then continued with phenytoin alone. The patient was transferred to the stroke unit. The objective neurological exam revealed the following data: the patient was awake, alert and interacting with his surroundings and with the doctor examining him; he presented global aphasia; he could carry out simple orders erratically, only by imitation and with a tendency to persist; he could raise his right arm a few centimetres from the bed; he could hold the Mingazzini II position on the right side. NIHSS = 16/42: 0-2-1-0-2-2-(0-2-0-0)-0-2-3-2-0. Anticoagulant therapy was reintroduced after approximately a month, when the CT results showed resolution of the haemorrhagic infarction.

2.6.1   Topics of Discussion

- Thrombolysis of a patient on NOACs: Which diagnostic tests? Which therapeutic approach?

  In literature there are only case reports on patients receiving therapy with rivaroxaban and dabigatran, treated with systemic fibrinolysis; there is still almost nothing on apixaban. In the absence of further data and while waiting to gain experience in the centres where thrombolysis is practised, it would be appropriate to limit thrombolytic treatment to carefully selected cases.
  Patient selection:

  1. Carry out brain CT scan and CT angiography to establish the location of the arterial occlusion.
  2. In patients with documented occlusion of the inside intracranial carotid, basilar artery or segments M1 or M2 of the middle cerebral artery, the therapeutic option to take into consideration is mechanical endovascular revascularization.

3. In patients with evidence of ischaemic stroke with no occlusion of a main arterial branch.

   (a) If the new anticoagulant is taken orally within 12–24 h of the event, venous thrombolysis can be considered.

       – With levels of the new oral anticoagulant below the limit of detection (10–30 ng/ml) determined through specific tests for the various DOAC
       – Or with aPTT within the norm if the patient takes dabigatran, or prothrombin time (PT) within the norm if the patient takes rivaroxaban or apixaban, and only after careful evaluation of the individual risk/benefit ratio (severity of the clinical picture, prognostic estimation of the treatment's possible success), variables which are normally correlated to a greater risk of haemorrhagic complications

   (b) If the new oral anticoagulant is taken orally within 48-h cerebral ischaemic event, there are no absolute contraindications for endovenous thrombolysis.

• What is the timing for resuming anticoagulant therapy?
  In patients with haemorrhagic infarction who have undergone decompression surgery (case study), the timing for reintroducing the anticoagulant drug is exactly the same as for patients with intraparenchymal haemorrhage.

2.7   Case Study No. 7

Presentation of the case of a 29-year-old woman. The patient was obese; she had been under oestrogen-progestin therapy for menstrual irregularities for 2 years. The patient arrived at the emergency department of a peripheral hospital (Spoke) because of the onset of paraesthesias of left hemiface and left arm. The symptoms started 12 h earlier and were followed by generalized tonic-clonic seizures. In the emergency department she was submitted to a brain CT scan without contrast, which showed a right hemispheric subarachnoid haemorrhage, signs of haemorrhagic infarction in the right frontal area and hypodense lesion of ischaemic origin in the left parietal region.

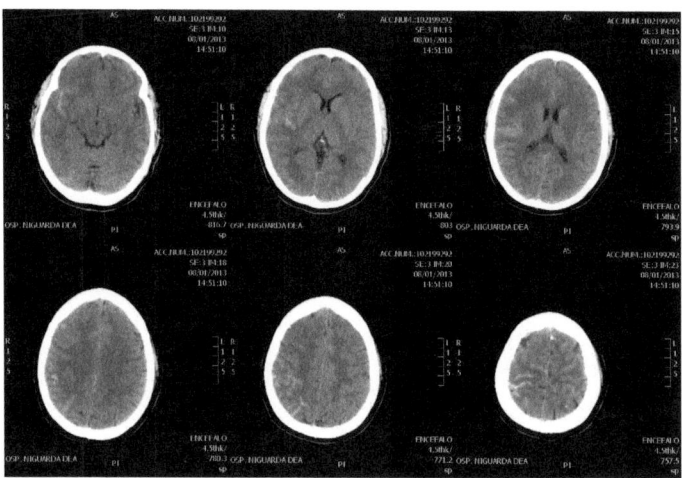

Brain CT scan results: right hemispheric subarachnoid haemorrhage, right frontal haemorrhagic infarction, and ischaemic hypodensity in the left parietal region.

Considering the complexity of the clinical and neuroradiological picture, the consequent need for complex neuroradiological investigations and dedicated instrumental monitoring, the patient was transferred to a high-complexity hospital (Hub) where neurologists, neurosurgeons, neuro-resuscitators, as well as high-profile diagnosis technologies and advanced therapeutic procedures were available. Upon admittance to the stroke unit, the patient was alert, cognitive motor slowing and oriented in time and space. She showed right deviation of gaze. The comparison test showed a disorder of the visual field: i.e., left lateral homonymous hemi-anopsia. Global strength tests after stroke showed poor alignment of the left upper limb. Examination of tactile sensitivity showed painful tactile hypoaesthesia of the left arm. The patient was anosognosic and showed hemi-inattention. NIHSS 7/42: 0-0-0-1-2-0-(1-0-0-0)-0-1-0-0-2. A CT angiography was performed which showed a thrombosis of the superior sagittal sinus, confirmed in MRI and venous angio-MRI carried out in urgency.

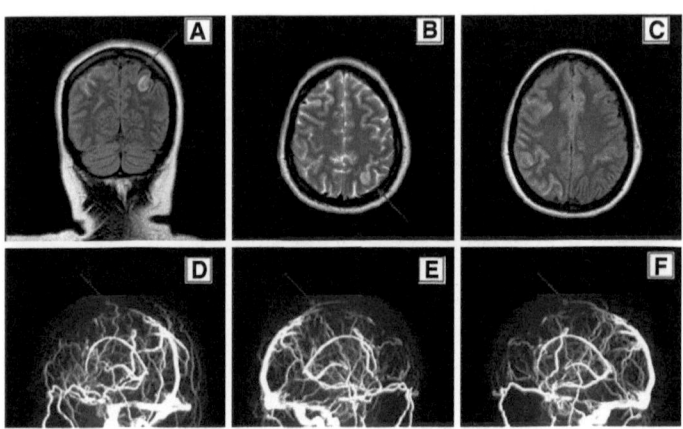

Brain MRI + venous angio-MRI: subarachnoid haemorrhage in some cortical sulci in the FLuid Attenuated Inversion Recovery (FLAIR) sequence (a and c) in addition to venous infarction in sequences T2 (b) and FLAIR (a). Three days venous reconstructions (d–f) did not show any opacity of the anterior portion of the upper sagittal sinus.

Given the nature of the clinical event (cerebral venous thrombosis), anticoagulant therapy with low molecular weight heparin (12,000 units) overlapped with oral anticoagulant therapy (warfarin) was started on the fourth day as well as the antiepileptic treatment with levetiracetam. Twenty-four hours after being transferred to the ward, the patient showed a clear clinical improvement and her NIHSS was 0/42. The patient was discharged with mRS = 0 and BI = 100/100. The results of a MRI performed 15 days after discharge showed an initial recanalization of the superior sagittal sinus and no residual signs of venous infarction.

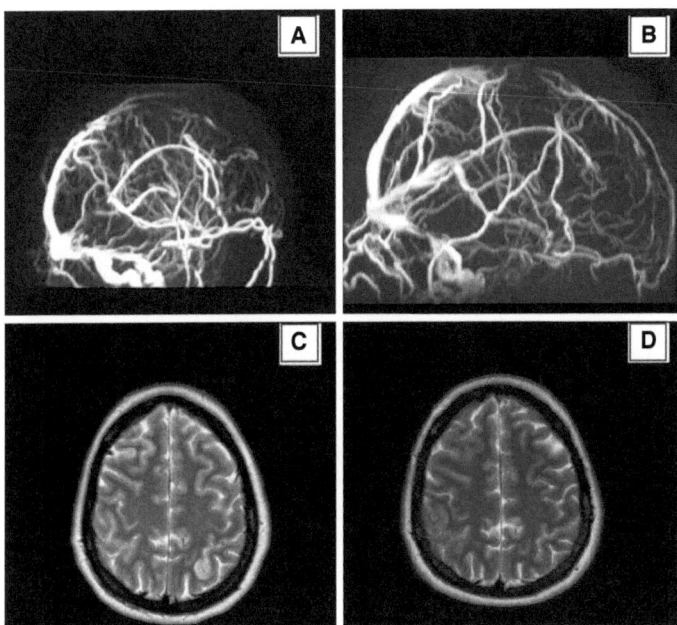

MRI + venous angio-MRI: partial occlusion of the superior sagittal sinus (a) with associated venous infarction (c). A test 15 days later showed an initial recanalization of the sagittal sinus (b) and almost complete disappearance of venous infarction (d).

2.7.1   Topics for Discussion

- Anticoagulant therapy in cerebral venous thrombosis: which and when?

  In case of an ascertained cerebral venous thrombosis, the anticoagulant therapy with intravenous heparin or low weight molecular heparin must immediately be delivered also to patients with evidence of ongoing cerebral haemorrhage. Data from literature show how anticoagulant therapy is associated with a significant reduction of mortality in patients affected by cerebral venous thrombosis, even in the presence of haemorrhagic infarction.

References

1. Vidale S, Beghi E, Gerardi F et al (2013) Time to hospital admission and start of treatment in patients with ischemic stroke in northern Italy and predictors of delay. Eur Neurol 70:349–355
2. Vidale S, Verrengia E, Gerardi F et al (2012) Stroke management in northern Lombardy: organization of an emergency-urgency network and development of a connection between prehospital and in-hospital settings. Int J Stroke 7(6):527–533
3. Vidale S, Agostoni E (2013) Time is brain: optimizing acute stroke management to reduce time delay. Acta Neurol Scand 127(3):e13–e14
4. Vidale S, Agostoni E (2014) Reducing the avoidable time in the management of stroke patients. Int J Cardiol 174(3):731
5. Vidale S, Agostoni E (2014) Thrombolysis in acute ischaemic stroke. Brain 137(6):e281
6. Imai K, Mori D, Izumoto H et al (2005) Emergency carotid artery stent placement in patients with acute ischemic stroke. AJNR 26:1249–1258
7. Jovin TG, Gupta R, Uchino K et al (2005) Emergency stenting of extracranial internal carotid artery occlusion has a high revascularization rate. Stroke 36:2426–2430
8. Nedeltchev K, Brekenfeld C, Remonda L et al (2005) Internal carotid artery stent implantation in 25 patients with acute stroke: preliminary results. Radiology 237:1029–1037
9. Nikas D, Reimers B, Elisabetta M et al (2007) Percutaneous interventions in patients with acute ischemic stroke related to obstructive atherosclerotic disease or dissection of the extracranial carotid artery. J Endovasc Ther 14:279–288

10. Zinkstok SM, Roos YB (2012) Early administration of aspirin in patients treated with alteplase for acute ischaemic stroke: a randomised controlled trial. Lancet 380:731–737
11. Karlinski M, Kobayashi A, Czlonkowska A et al (2014) Role of preexisting disability in patients treated with intravenous thrombolysis for ischemic stroke. Stroke 45(3):770–775

Chapter 3
Organizational Clinical Pathways

Valentina Oppo, Cristina Motto, and Valentina Perini

All patients with stroke or suspected stroke benefit from integrated stroke care systems which are created following the recommendations in the guidelines of the American Heart Association (AHA)/American Stroke Association (ASA) [1]. These care systems include hospitals for treating acute stroke, which often offer telemedicine and teleradiology, comprehensive stroke units, emergency units, public agencies and government resources. The objectives are prevention of stroke, optimal use of emergency departments, treatment of acute and subacute stroke, rehabilitation and follow-up, as well as educational programmes. Randomized clinical trials have shown that patients treated in primary stroke centres have a better outcome than patients treated in facilities without a stroke unit and that the rate of thrombolysis is higher; thus in the AHA/ASA guidelines, the creation of primary stroke centres is recommended (Class I, Evidence Level B), pointing out that these centres must be certified by an external organization. They further recommend setting up a multidisciplinary "improvement and quality" commission for reviewing and monitoring quality indicators, such as quality of care, evidence-based practice and prognosis (Class I, Level of Evidence B), in order to identify any deficiencies and to arrange to have them corrected.

The organization of resources depends on what local resources are available. Patients with suspected stroke should be sent to the nearest stroke unit: hospitals without such units should be avoided. For those care centres that do not have

G. D'Aliberti et al., *Ischemic Stroke*, Emergency Management in Neurology, DOI 10.1007/978-3-319-31705-2_3,
© Springer International Publishing Switzerland 2017

specific competence in the interpretation of neuroimaging, development of a teleradiology system is recommended in order to read the images quickly, thus enabling rapid decisions about fibrinolytic therapy. The creation of comprehensive stroke care units (Class I, Level of Evidence C) which can treat stroke 24 h a day/7 days a week is also recommended. Such care units include neuro-intensive care units. Clinical studies have shown that in these units there is no difference in the rate of mortality and prognosis in reference to the moment of admittance (i.e. weekend) and that prognosis is associated with the structural and professional complexity of the centre. Facilities without specific competences for stroke care should implement a system of teleconsultation associated with educational programmes and personnel training in order to increase the delivery of thrombolytic therapy (Class IIa, Level of Evidence B). The creation of hospitals ready to receive patients with suspected stroke might be useful even if they do not have internal stroke units. Such hospitals should have a protocol for stroke care in emergency, perform thrombolysis and be closely associated with facilities which have a comprehensive care system that can deliver extensive and complete treatments (Class IIa, Level of Evidence C).

3.1   Clinical Evaluation in Emergency

In the presence of a patient with suspected ischaemic stroke who is potentially eligible for reperfusion therapy, clinical assessment should be targeted at identifying and excluding possible conditions similar to stroke (so-called stroke mimics) and at establishing the time of onset of symptoms [1], which is the main criterion for a patient being eligible for reperfusion treatment, as well as the main factor that may limit the effectiveness of the treatment itself [2–4]. When the time of onset of symptoms is unknown, it is conventionally traced back to the last time the patient was seen to be healthy. When the symptoms of stroke are already present on awakening, the time of onset is traced back to the time the patient went to bed [1]. The clinical neurological evaluation must be carried out using the NIHSS [5]. According to AHA/ASA guidelines, the blood tests to be performed in the acute phase are glycaemia, renal function, blood count with platelets, cardiac enzymes, PT (prothrombin time), INR and PTT (partial thromboplastin time) [1]. For patients who are not on anticoagulation therapy or do not show any signs of thrombocytopenia, coagulopathy or liver disease, it is not necessary to wait for the results of the blood counts and coagulation tests before starting reperfusion treatment, as the incidence of non-suspected coagulopathy is very low, less than 1 % [6, 7]. This recommendation is not confirmed in the European guidelines by the European Stroke Organization (ESO) nor in the latest edition of the SPREAD guidelines of 2012 [8, 9]. On the contrary, it is absolutely necessary to acquire the value of capillary blood glucose (CBG) because symptomatic hypoglycaemia is one of the potential stroke mimics. Furthermore, measurement of O_2 saturation is recommended, as is its correction with O_2 supplementation, if the patient is hypoxemic as well as the acquisition of electrocardiogram and blood pressure measurement.

3.2 Neuroimaging

An urgent CT brain scan without contrast medium can provide the informations necessary to develop therapeutic decisions [1]. This concept was confirmed in the updating of AHA/ASA guidelines on endovascular therapy, which was published in June 2015 [10]. In fact, although brain MRI has more sensitivity and more specificity in detecting acute ischaemic lesions than CT brain scan because of its higher resolution (especially on the structures of the posterior fossa) and the possibility of using DWI which can detect acute ischaemic lesions at a very early stage [11], it is an exam that takes time and cannot be performed on patients carrying pacemakers or other metallic devices. Furthermore, MRI is more sensitive to motion artefacts; it is less likely to be tolerated, especially by agitated or confused patients [1]; and it is not always available in urgency. The presence of early signs of ischaemia detected by means of a CT brain scan without contrast must not be a contraindication to intravenous reperfusion therapy because, even if signs are visible, the patient can still benefit from the treatment. Consideration must however be taken of the extent of the early signs of ischaemia: >1/3 of the territory of the middle cerebral artery (MCA) increases the risk of haemorrhage [12, 13]. The recommendations of the AHA/ASA guidelines state that early signs of ischaemia (if time of onset of symptoms is certain) must never be a reason for not delivering intravenous reperfusion therapy, unless a "clear hypodensity" is present, extending >1/3 of the territory of MCA [1]. An easy method of reading a CT scan without contrast, in order to determine the extension of an early ischaemic lesion, is the ASPECTS score [14]. The involvement of 1/3 of MCA territory corresponds to an ASPECTS score = ≤7. A non-invasive intracranial vascular neuroimaging CT angiogram needs to be performed when endovascular therapy is recommended, but it must not delay the administration of intravenous thrombolysis. CT or MRI perfusion techniques are indicated to detect ischaemic penumbra in special situations, primarily to assess the existence of a potential benefit from reperfusion therapy in patients with symptom onset outside the therapeutic window or when the time of symptom onset is uncertain (recommendation Level C according to AHA/ASA guidelines). The AHA/ASA, ESO and ISO guidelines agree on the fact that if the patient has an onset of symptoms that can be set with certainty within the therapeutic window, it is not necessary to search for ischaemic penumbra because it makes no contribution to the decision-making strategy. The AHA/ASA guidelines outline an ideal timing to be observed in the different stages of clinical and instrumental evaluations of acute stroke patients:

- Assessment by the emergency department doctor within 10 min
- Assessment by the stroke team within 15 min
- Performance of CT scan within 25 min

- Interpretation of CT brain scan within 45 min
- Start of thrombolytic therapy within 60 min (for at least 80 % of the patients)
- Admission to stroke unit within 3 h

3.3   Indications for Intravenous Reperfusion Therapy

Intravenous reperfusion treatment with alteplase is indicated for acute ischaemic stroke (dosage 0.9 mg/kg, maximum 90 mg, of which 10 % administered initially as a bolus and the remaining quantity over a period of 60 min). According to the results of the NINDS study [15], the therapeutic window (time from onset of symptoms) within which intravenous thrombolytic treatment can be delivered was originally 3 h. The data analysis of subsequent trials, such as ECASS III and IST-3 [16], showed that treating patients within 3–4.5 h of onset of symptoms gives a more modest clinical benefit than early treatment against a small increased risk of bleeding. When more than 4.5 h have elapsed from onset of symptoms, the clinical benefit is not significant [2–4, 16, 17]; for this reason the therapeutic window was extended to 4.5 h from symptom onset. The FDA (Food and Drug Administration), in contrast to EMA (European Medicines Agency) and AIFA (Agenzia Italiana del Farmaco), has not accepted the extension of the therapeutic window to 4.5 h. Thus AHA/ASA guidelines, unlike ESO and ISO guidelines, assign an indication of Level B and not of Level A to the administration of alteplase for treatment of acute stroke within 4.5 h, with the recommendation that a more restrictive approach be adopted regarding the other criteria if the thrombolytic is administered between 3 and 4.5 h [1]. All the guidelines agree on recommending administration of the drug as early as possible, given the inverse linear relation existing between the efficacy of reperfusion therapy and the time the therapy is administered [18]. The AHA/ASA guidelines indicate a precise timing: the therapy should be delivered within 60 min from the patient's arrival at the emergency department. According to AHA/ASA, the absolute exclusion criteria for intravenous thrombolytic therapy are as follows:

- Age below 18 years.
- Recent severe trauma or stroke in the last 3 months. According to the most recent updating of Italian guidelines by the ISO, dated March 2015, stroke in the previous 3 months actually represents a relative contraindication, to be assessed according to time, extension of the previous stroke, age of the patient (the older the patient, the higher the risk of bleeding and the shorter the life expectancy) and potential severity of the ongoing event.
- Puncture of a noncompressible blood vessel (<7 days).
- History of intracranial haemorrhage.
- Neoplasms, aneurysm or intracranial arteriovenous malformation.
- Recent major intracranial or spinal neurosurgery.
- Blood pressure >185/110 mmHg.

According to 2012 SPREAD guidelines, if more than one intravenous administration of antihypertensive is needed to reach the therapeutic blood pressure target, this is a contraindication to administrating alteplase. In the update of ISO recommendations dated March 2015 [19], it is stated that the therapy is in any case indicated once the therapeutic target has been achieved. No limitations are mentioned regarding the therapy needed in order to reach the therapeutic target.

- Severe active or recent bleeding (last 3 months).
- Haemorrhagic diathesis, along with but not only: platelet count inferior to $100,000/mm^3$; intravenous administration of heparin in the last 48 h and aPTT values exceeding the upper limit; administration of warfarin with INR >1.7 or PT >15 s; use of direct thrombin or Xa factor inhibitor drugs with significant alteration in laboratory test values (aPTT, INR, platelet count, ecarin time, TT) or in other specific tests of Xa factor activity. Intravenous thromboly-

sis is indicated if the patient has not been on anticoagulant therapy with direct thrombin or Xa factor inhibitor drugs for at least 2 days and renal function is not altered. Patients who do not use oral anticoagulants or heparin, and who are not known for haemorrhagic diathesis, can start receiving thrombolytic treatment before blood test results are available. Such treatment will be interrupted if PT becomes longer or a thrombocytemia value of below 100,000/mm^3 emerges.

Regarding therapy with Warfarin, new ISO recommendations from March 2015 agree on the indication of thrombolytic therapy, provided that PT INR is ≤1.7, while EMA recommendations contraindicate the use of thrombolytic even with subtherapeutic INR, provided it is over the normal range. It has been demonstrated that patients on OAT (oral anticoagulant therapy) with subtherapeutic INR who receive intravenous thrombolysis are more likely to suffer a symptomatic haemorrhagic transformation of the ischaemic lesion, but there is no evidence of worse outcome or increased mortality when compared to patients who are not treated with warfarin [20]. However, with patients on anticoaugulants and who have INR ≤1.7, AHA/ASA guidelines restrict the indication of therapy to administration within 3 h from onset of symptoms. With patients on anticoagulant therapy, thrombolytic therapy is always contraindicated between 3 and 4.5 h. This restriction is not mentioned in the Italian guidelines. As for heparin therapy, EMA and AIFA indications are in line with AHA/ASA guidelines (contraindication in patients who have received heparin therapy in the previous 48 h, with altered aPTT); the SPREAD guidelines from 2012 restrict contraindication to 24 h before the event, without mentioning the aPTT value. As regards indication of thrombolytic therapy during treatment with new oral anticoagulants, the 2012 SPREAD guidelines are in line with AHA/ASA guidelines which emphasize the need for negative results in specific tests which can assess the activities of the NOACs, in order to enable administration of a thrombolytic drug.

- Glycaemia below 50 mg/dl. The 2015 update of ISO recommendations [19] mentions the possibility of treating patients whose focal neurological deficit does not change after correcting glycaemia (Evidence Level GPP [good practice point]). Hyperglycaemia is not specifically mentioned as a contraindication to the treatment. According to the latest update of ISO guidelines [19], when glycaemia is >400 mg/dl, thrombolytic treatment is recommended if glycaemia decreases to <200 mg/dl within 4.5 h from onset of symptoms (Evidence Level GPP).
- Hypodensity on CT brain scan extending to >1/3 of MCA territory.

According to EMA and AIFA recommendations, there are further contraindications to intravenous administration of thrombolytic drug which are not directly connected to its use in treating ischaemic acute stroke, but to its general use:

- Strong suspicion of a subarachnoid haemorrhage even when bleeding does not appear on the CT scan (i.e. in the presence of strong headache and stiff neck)
- Haemorrhagic retinopathy caused by diabetes
- Recent (less than 10 days) external traumatic cardiac massage or delivery
- Bacterial endocarditis and pericarditis
- Acute pancreatitis
- Ulcerous disease of the gastrointestinal tract in the last 3 months, oesophageal varices, arterial aneurysm and arterial or venous malformations
- Neoplasms with increased risk of haemorrhage
- Severe hepatopathy, including hepatic insufficiency, cirrhosis, portal hypertension and active hepatitis (oesophageal varices)
- Recent major surgery or recent severe trauma (<3 months)
- According to AHA/ASA guidelines, the time limit is 14 days

AHA/ASA guidelines include some "relative" contraindications, which were originally absolute and have subsequently been revised on the basis of data derived from clinical experience and trials carried out after NINDS:

- Mild impairment or rapidly improving impairment: this contraindication was revised with reference to the fact that in an aphasic or hemianoptic or with strength impairment, a low NIHSS score can also be particularly disabling and with reference to some other studies that have shown how some patients with mild impairment at onset of symptoms and who were therefore not treated with thrombolytic therapy often had a negative outcome [21–23]. The recently updated ISO guidelines [19] confirm recommendation for thrombolytic treatment in patients with mild impairment or rapid improvement, provided that it is still detectable when treatment is started (recommendation B).
- Pregnancy: alteplase does not pass through the placenta because of its molecular size, it therefore has no teratogenic effects; the most serious risk is placenta abruption, and most of the cases reported in literature had a positive outcome [24]. Therefore, the administration of alteplase in pregnancy remains an off-label option to be assessed case by case on the basis of the risk/benefit ratio.
- Seizures at onset of symptoms: in this case treatment is indicated when there is clinical evidence that seizure is a consequence of focal deficit and is not a post-critical status. According to new ISO recommendations, it is possible to use neuroimaging and CT angiogram alongside clinical criteria to highlight occlusion of an intracranial vessel; MRI with DWI sequences to highlight an acute ischaemic lesion (GPP recommendations).
- Recent bleeding in the gastrointestinal or urinary tract (in the previous 21 days).
- Recent acute myocardial infarct (AMI) (in the last 3 months): in this case the indication is justified by the potential risk of intracardiac bleeding, but depending on assessment of the risk/benefit ratio, it is however possible to deliver therapy.

The upper age limit of 80 years is no longer mentioned in AHA/ASA and ISO recommendations. In fact, the patients in this age group still benefit significantly from intravenous thrombolytic therapy [4, 16, 18]. For the same reason, according to the results of IST-3 which were confirmed in the meta-analysis of patient's individual data deriving from randomized studies [18], the upper severity limit of the contraindication has been eliminated (NIHSS >25), because it has been proven that these patients still benefit from reperfusion therapy [4].

The updating of the ISO guidelines dated March 2015 explicitly states that recommendation for administering intravenous reperfusion therapy with alteplase within 4.5 h from onset of symptoms does not have any upper age or severity limit (recommendation Level A).

Both in the ISO and AHA/ASA guidelines, the contraindication for patients with previous stroke and diabetes has been removed.

Upper age or severity limits, stroke and diabetes mellitus as well as oral anticoagulant therapy independently of INR values are still valid contraindications in AHA/ASA guidelines for patients treated between 3 and 4.5 h. This is because, when faced with the risk/benefit ratio, it was considered adequate to select patients with better profiles in terms of other factors which are predictive of the treatment results. However, this restriction is not mentioned in the ESO and ISO guidelines.

The following are the AHA/ASA guideline indications for management during treatment with intravenous thrombolysis and the post-treatment phase:

- Admit to stroke unit for monitoring of vital parameters.
- Pay special attention to the development of orolingual angioedema that can cause obstruction of the airways. It is generally a transient and mild reaction, reported in approximately 5 % of the patients treated, and its risk increases with the use of ACE inhibitors [25].
- Measure blood pressure and assess patient's neurological status every 15 min during intravenous thrombolysis and

in the 2 h following it, then every 30 min for 6 h and then every 60 min for 24 h.

- If the patient presents headache, nausea, vomiting and worsening of neurological conditions, thrombolytic treatment (if in progress) should be interrupted and a CT brain scan should be performed to exclude the risk of intracranial haemorrhage.
- If blood pressure exceeds 180/105 mmHg in the 24 h following thrombolysis, blood pressure must be measured more frequently, and the patient must be treated with intravenous agents to keep blood pressure under the values mentioned above.
- If possible, defer insertion of urinary catheter, nasogastric tube or intra-arterial catheter to monitor blood pressure.
- Do not administer either anticoagulants or antiplatelet agents within the first 24 h after thrombolysis. These can be administered after assessing the CT scan after reperfusion therapy. This indication was in the original NINDS protocol [15]. It was subsequently shown that co-administration of streptokinase and acetylsalicylic acid (ASA) in acute stroke increases mortality, most likely because of an increase in the risk of haemorrhage [17, 26]. This recommendation is still valid since there are no studies demonstrating the safety and benefit of administrating ASA soon after thrombolytic therapy [1].

3.4   Indications for Endovascular Therapy

In June 2015 an update of the 2013 AHA/ASA guidelines was published, regarding endovascular treatment in the acute phase of stroke. The update included the results of eight trials on endovascular therapy in the acute stroke phase, the results of which were published between 2013 and 2015 [10]: SYNTHESIS, IMS III, MR RESCUE, MR CLEAN, ESCAPE, SWIFT PRIME, EXTEND IA and REVASCAT.

Level "A" indication for endovascular therapy was given to patients over 18 years of age, starting from a good neurological status (mRS pre-event 0 or 1), with occlusion of the internal carotid artery or of the proximal segment (M1) of the MCA, with an NIHSS score of ≥6 and an ASPECTS score of ≥6 [14]. These restrictions are due to the fact that most of the trials were carried out on selected patients who had these character-istics; thus data are not sufficient to determine whether clinical benefit is preserved also in patients with a more serious clinical status or for patients with early ischaemic signs which are more extensive.

Puncture of the arterial vessel can be performed up to 6 h from onset of symptoms. This time limit is linked to the fact that the thrombectomy procedure could be started within 6 h for most of the patients involved in these trials and that data regarding patients treated within 8 and 12 h, which were col-lected in REVASCAT and ESCAPE [27, 28], were insufficient to determine the effectiveness in this time window. Furthermore, sub-analysis of MR CLEAN results showed that when therapy was started later than 6 h from onset of symptoms, patients did not significantly benefit from the treatment [29].

All patients who are eligible for endovenous thrombolysis must first be treated with this therapy. Contrary to what was stated in the 2013 guidelines, indication for endovascular therapy is not limited to patients who are unresponsive to endovenous therapy; in fact, it is explicitly stated that it is not necessary to observe the patients and candidate them for endovascular treatment only if they do not improve with intravenous treatment. If the patients have criteria which make them eligible for endovascular therapy, they must be treated as soon as possible. In fact, as regards intravenous treatment, the best results are obtained by treating patients as early as possible [29, 30]. Similarly, it is not necessary to repeat CT angiography to confirm arterial occlusion before starting endovascular treatment. In fact this strategy was used in REVASCAT, and there was no evidence of better clinical results [28]. The indication for endovascular therapy is Level C in patients with occlusion of distal segments of the MCA (M2 or M3), anterior cerebral arteries (ACA), posterior cere-bral arteries (PCA) and vertebral or basilar arteries. The same level (C) is also assigned to endovascular therapy for patients aged <18 years and for patients who cannot be treated with endovenous thrombolysis because of specific contraindications.

Finally, a Level C recommendation is assigned to angioplasty and/or stenting treatment in acute stenosis of cervical tract of carotid artery when thrombectomy is performed.

The March 2015 update of ISO recommendations highlights that if endovenous thrombolytic treatment is indicated, there is no alternative treatment [19]. Evidence Level B is assigned to endovascular treatment of stroke with internal carotid occlusion, MCA in segments M1 and M2 and ACA in the proximal segment that do not respond to, or do not have any indications for, intravenous thrombolysis.

When there is an occlusion of major vessels of the posterior circulation (vertebral, basilar, cerebral arteries in the proximal segment), a GPP indication level is assigned to endovascular treatment on patients who do not respond to or do not have any indications for endovenous thrombolytic treatment.

ESO guidelines, which were published in 2008 and therefore are not based on the results of recent trials on endovascular therapy, assign a Level B recommendation to endovascular treatment of MCA occlusion within 6 h from onset of symptoms, and of basilar artery beyond 3 h, without time limits.

3.5 Monitoring Vital Signs of the Patient in the Stroke Unit

An integral part of the best therapy for acute stroke, regardless of whether reperfusion therapy is delivered, is the treatment of the patient in a stroke unit [1]. If the patient is not administered endovenous thrombolysis, blood pressure values have a higher limit in the first 24 h: treatment is recommended when blood pressure values exceed 220/120 mmHg, unless coexisting medical conditions other than stroke are likely to be exacerbated by high blood pressure (AMI, heart failure, aortic dissection). AHA/ASA, ESO and ISO guidelines agree on this indication, and the rationale lies in the demonstration of an unfavourable outcome either in the case of hypertension or hypotension, with greater benefit to moderate hypertension [31, 32]. AHA/ASA guidelines recommend monitoring body temperature and treating hyperthermia. It has been proven that increased body temperature is associated with doubling short-term mortality [33]. The recent ESO focus on body temperature management of acute stroke patients has shown that there is no firm evidence of a better outcome in terms of mortality and independence through the symptomatic treatment of hyperthermic patients with antipyretics nor by using antipyretics to prevent hyperthermia in normothermic patients. It remains an indication of good clinical practice to prevent and treat underlying infections and hyperthermia as a symptom, in order to avoid discomfort for the patient [34]. Monitoring of oximetry and correction of any possible hypoxaemia is recommended (in AHA/ASA guidelines if saturimetry falls below 94 %, in SPREAD guidelines if saturimetry falls below 92 %). Hyperglycaemia is associated with a higher rate of intracranial haemorrhage and with a worse outcome in patients with acute stroke [35, 36]; it is therefore necessary to monitor and control glycaemia values pharmacologically if they are high, but trials on the treatment of glycaemia in the acute stroke phase have not shown any improvement in outcome for patients treated [37]; thus an optimal target for glycaemia values has never been identified. At the moment, therefore, reference is made to the American Diabetes Association guidelines [38], which recommend maintaining the glycaemia values of all hospitalized patients at between 140 and 180 mg/dl. Again, on the basis of the negative effects of hyperglycaemia in the first phases of stroke, administration of glucose solutions is not recommended for intravenous hydration of patients in the stroke unit: it would be preferable to administer saline solution.

According to AHA/ASA and ESO guidelines, continuous monitoring of heart rhythm is recommended for 24 h after hospitalization. Application of a Holter electrocardiogram (ECG) is also recommended if monitoring has shown no potentially cardioembolic arrhythmias and cardioembolic etiopathogenesis is still strongly suspected.

3.6   Management of Transient Ischaemic Attack

AHA/ASA guidelines recommend that patients presenting at the emergency department with TIA should undergo a neuroimaging examination within 24 h from onset of symptoms and in any case as early as possible. Brain MRI is referred to as the most suitable method because it can identify recent small ischaemic areas. If no MRI can be performed in urgency, then a CT brain scan is sufficient. The 2008 ESO guidelines agree on this point, but do not indicate any specific timing within which neuroradiological investigations must be performed. The reason for neuroimaging investigation in the acute phase is that the patients with ischaemic lesions are more likely to suffer a further ischaemic event, possibly more disabling in the short term. The risks of a stroke or a minor stroke within 7 days after TIA are, respectively, 8 % and 12 % [39]. In any case, the clinical scores used to quantify the risk of early recurrence (e.g. ABCD) are as critically important as imaging [40].

Furthermore, a study of extracranial vessels is recommended with colour Doppler of supra-aortic trunks as part of assessment in urgency. According to the indications of the 2008 ESO guidelines, a Doppler must be considered a priority in the case of a TIA, more than in the case of a stroke with large ischaemic lesions. This is because if there is an ipsilateral carotid stenosis on the side of the vascular event, the TIA patient can benefit from surgery in the short term, which is not true for patients with large ischaemic lesions.

Furthermore, ECG and blood tests are recommended for ischaemic stroke.

The ESO guidelines highlight the need for continuous monitoring of ECG for TIA patients, whereas the recommendation in AHA/ASA guidelines refers only to stroke patients.

The 2012 SPREAD guidelines are basically in line with AHA/ASA and ESO guidelines in recommending that neuroimaging investigations be carried out in urgency, preferably an MRI because it offers higher resolution in the study of posterior fossa, as well as Doppler ultrasound of supra-aortic trunks, ECG and blood tests. All necessary investigations must be completed within 48 h from admittance to the emergency department. As for continuous monitoring of ECG, it is not explicitly recommended for TIA patients (who need hospitalization only if they reach ABCD2 ≥4). A Holter ECG study is recommended in the acute phase if there is a strong suspicion that the stroke is of cardioembolic origin.

3.7   Management of Acute Complications of Ischaemic Stroke

Cerebral oedema develops in 1–10 % of supratentorial stroke patients, generally from 2 to 5 days from onset [41, 42], but in approximately one third of the cases, it develops in the first 24 h, especially when there is early reperfusion of a large portion of necrotic tissue [43]. Both AHA/ASA and ESO guidelines assign an indication of Level C to the use of osmotic drugs (glycerol and mannitol) to reduce cerebral oedema. Administration of intravenous corticosteroid is contraindicated.

Neither prophylactic antiepileptic therapy nor prophylactic antibiotic therapy is recommended [44]. Stronger recommendations (Level A for ESO guidelines, Level B for AHA/ASA guidelines) are assigned to decompressive craniectomy for hemispheric oedema in selected patients: under 60 years of age, with clinical and radiological evidence of an important involvement of the MCA territory and deterioration of consciousness. This procedure is recommended within 48 h from the event [41]. Both in AHA/ASA and in ESO guidelines, despite the lack of trials on the topic and therefore recommendation Level C, surgical decompression or ventriculostomy is strongly recommended in patients with ischaemia of posterior fossa, by virtue of the favourable clinical outcome associated with this procedure, even for patients who are comatose before the event [45].

Haemorrhagic Transformation: in patients receiving intravenous thrombolysis, the rate of symptomatic haemorrhagic transformation is between 5 and 6 % [46]. There are no specific guidelines on haemorrhagic transformation in fibrinolysis; thus reference must be made to guidelines on spontaneous intraparenchymal haemorrhage.

References

1. Jauch EC, Saver JL, Adams HP et al (2013) Guidelines for the early management of patients with acute ischemic stroke. A guideline for healthcare professionals from the American Heart Association/American Stroke Association. Stroke 44:870–947
2. Kennedy RL, Bluhmki E, Von Kummer R et al (2010) Time to treatment with intravenous alteplase and outcome in stroke: an updated pooled analysis of ECASS, ATLANTIS, NINDS and EPITHET trials. Lancet 375:1695–1703
3. Saver JL, Fonarow JC, Smith EE et al (2013) Time to treatment with intravenous tissue plasminogen activator and outcome from acute ischemic stroke. JAMA 309(23):2480–2488
4. Wardlaw JM, Murray V, Berge E et al (2012) Recombinant Tissue Plasminogen Activator for acute ischaemic stroke: an updated systematic review and meta-analysis. Lancet 379: 2364–2372
5. Josephson SA, Hills NK, Johnston SC (2006) NIH stroke scale reliability in ratings from a large sample of clinicians. Cerebrovasc Dis 22:389–395
6. Rost NS, Masrur S, Pervez MA et al (2009) Unsuspected coagulopathy rarely prevents IV thrombolysis in acute ischemic stroke. Neurology 73:1957–1962
7. Cucchiara BL, Jackson B, Weiner M et al (2007) Usefulness of checking platelet count before thrombolysis in acute ischemic stroke. Stroke 38:1639–1640
8. European Stroke Organization (ESO) Executive Committee, ESO Writing Committee (2008) Guidelines for management of ischaemic stroke and transient ischemic attack. Cerebrovasc Dis 25:457–507

9. Stroke Prevention And Educational Awareness Diffusion (SPREAD). Ictus cerebrale: linee guida italiane di prevenzione e trattamento. VII edizione. Stesura del 14 marzo 2012.

10. Powers WJ, Derdeyn CP, Biller J et al (2015) 2015 AHA/ASA focused update of the 2013 guidelines for the early management of patients with acute ischemic stroke regarding endovascular treatment. Stroke 46:3020–3035

11. Barber PA, Darby DG, Desmond PM et al (1999) Identification of major ischemic change: diffusion-weighted imaging versus computed tomography. Stroke 30(10):2059–2065

12. Larrue V, Von Kummer R, Del Zoppo G et al (1997) Hemorrhagic transformation in acute ischemic stroke: potential contributing factors in European Cooperative Acute Stroke Study. Stroke 28:957–960

13. Patel SC, Levine SR, Tilley BC et al (2001) National Institute of Neurological Disorders and Stroke rt-PA Stroke Study Group. Lack of significance of early ischemic stroke on computed tomography in acute stroke. JAMA 286:2830–2838

14. Pexman JH, Barber PA, Hill MD et al (2001) Use of the Alberta Stroke Program Early CT Score (ASPECTS) for assessing CT scans in patients with acute stroke. AJNR 22:1534–1542

15. The National Institute of Neurological Disorders and Stroke rt-PA Study Group (1995) Tissue plasminogen activator for acute ischemic stroke. N Engl J Med 333:1581–1587

16. Sandercock P, Wardlaw JM, Lindley RI et al (2012) The benefits and harms of intravenous thrombolysis with recombinant tissue plasminogen activator within 6 h of acute ischaemic stroke (the third international stroke trial [IST-3]): a randomized controlled trial. Lancet Neurol 379:2352–2363

17. Wardlaw JM, Murray V, Berge E et al (2014) Thrombolysis for acute ischemic stroke. Cochrane Database Syst Rev 7:CD000213

18. Emberson J, Lees KR, Lyden P et al. for the Stroke Thrombolysis Trialists' Collaborative Group (2014) Effect of treatment delay, age, and stroke severity on the effects of intravenous thrombolysis with alteplase for acute ischaemic stroke: a meta-analysis of individual patient data from randomised trials. Lancet 384:1929–1935

19. Toni D, Mangiafico S, Agostoni E et al (2015) Intravenous thrombolysis and intra-arterial interventions in acute ischemic stroke: Italian Stroke Organisation (ISO)-SPREAD guidelines. Int J Stroke 10:1119–1129

20. Miedema I, Luijckx GJ, De Keyser J et al (2012) Thrombolytic therapy for ischaemic stroke in patients using warfarin: a systematic review and meta-analysis. J Neurol Neurosurg Psychiatry 83:537–540

21. De Keyser I, Gdovinovà Z, Uyttenboogaart M et al (2007) Intravenous alteplase for stroke: beyond the guidelines and in particular clinical situations. Stroke 38:2612–2618

22. Smith EE, Abdullah AR, Petkovska I et al (2005) Poor outcomes in patients who do not receive intravenous tissue plasminogen activator because of mild or improving ischemic stroke. Stroke 36:2497–2499

23. Tong DC (2012) Avoiding thrombolysis in patients with mild stroke: is it SMART? Stroke 43(3):625–626

24. Tassi R, Acampa M, Marotta G et al (2013) Systemic thrombolysis for stroke in pregnancy. Am J Emerg Med 31(2):448.e1–448.e3

25. Hill MD, Lye T, Moss H et al (2003) Hemi-orolingual angioedema and ACE inhibition after alteplase treatment of stroke. Neurology 60:1525–1527

26. Ciccone A, Motto C, Aritzu E et al (2000) Negative interaction of aspirin and streptokinase in acute ischemic stroke: further analysis of the Multicenter Acute Stroke Trial-Italy. Cerebrovasc Dis 10(1):61–64

27. Goyal M, Demchuk AM, Menon BK et al (2015) Randomized assessment of rapid endovascular treatment of ischemic stroke. N Engl J Med 372:1019–1030

28. Jovin TG, Chamorro A, Cobo E et al (2015) Thrombectomy within 8 hours after symptom on onset in ischemic stroke. N Engl J Med 372:2296–2306

29. Fransen P, Berkhemer O, Lingsma H, Beumer D, van den Berg L, van Zwam W, van Oostenbrugge R, van der Lugt A, Majoie C, Dippel D, for the MR CLEAN Investigators (2016) Time to reperfusion and effect of intra-arterial treatment in the MR CLEAN Trial. JAMA Neurol 73(2):190–196

30. Prabahakaran S, Ruff I, Bernstein RA (2015) Acute stroke intervention: a systematic review. JAMA 313(14):1451–1462

31. Okumura K, Ohya Y, Maehara A et al (2005) Effects of blood pressure levels on case fatality after acute stroke. J Hypertens 23:1217–1223

32. Leonardi-Bee J, Bath PM, Phillips SJ (2002) Blood pressure and clinical outcomes in international stroke trial. Stroke 33:1315–1320

33. Prasad K, Krishnan PR (2010) Fever is associated with doubling of odds of short term mortality in ischemic stroke: an updated meta-analysis. Acta Neurol Scand 122:404–408

34. Ntaios G, Dziedzic T, Michel P et al (2015) European Stroke Organization (ESO) guidelines for the management of temperature in patients with acute ischemic stroke. Int J Stroke 10(6):941–949

35. Bruno A, Levine SR, Frankel MR et al (2002) Admission glucose level and clinical outcomes in the NINDS rt-PA stroke trial. Neurology 59:669–674

36. Demchuk AM, Tanne D, Hill MD et al (2001) Predictors of good outcome after intravenous tPA for acute ischemic stroke. Neurology 57:474–480

37. Bellolio MF, Gilmore RM, Ganti L (2014) Insulin for Glycaemic control in acute ischaemic stroke. Cochrane Database Syst Rev 9:CD005346

38. American Diabetes Association (2010) Standard of medical care in diabetes. Diabetes Care 33:692

39. Coull AJ, Lovett JK, Rothwell PM et al (2004) Population based study of early risk of stroke after transient ischemic attack or minor stroke: implication for public education and organization of services. BMJ 328(7435):326

40. Redgrave JN, Coutts SB, Schulz UG et al (2007) Systematic review of association between the presence of acute ischemic lesion on diffusion-weighted imaging and clinical predictors of early stroke risk after transient ischemic attack. Stroke 38:1482–1488

41. Vahedi K, Hofmeijer J, Juettler E et al (2007) Early decompressive surgery in malignant infarction of the middle cerebral artery: a pooled analysis of three randomized controlled trials. Lancet Neurol 6:215–222

42. Qureshy AI, Suarez JI, Yahia AM et al (2003) Timing of neurological deterioration in massive middle cerebral artery infarction: a multicenter review. Crit Care Med 31:272–277

43. Hacke W, Schwab S, Horn M (1996) "Malignant" middle cerebral artery territory infarction: clinical course and prognostic signs. Arch Neurol 53:309–315

44. Westendorp WF, Vermeij JD, Zock E et al. for the PASS investigators (2015) The Preventive Antibiotics in Stroke Study (PASS): a pragmatic randomized open-label masked endpoint clinical trial. Lancet 385:1519–1526

45. Chen HJ, Lee TC, Wei CP (1992) Treatment of cerebellar infarction by decompressive suboccipital craniectomy. Stroke 23:957–961
46. Leigh R, Zaidat OO, Suri MF et al (2004) Predictors of hyperacute clinical worsening in ischemic stroke patients receiving thrombolytic therapy. Stroke 35:1903–1907

Chapter 4
Differentiated Decisional Algorithms

Simone Vidale, Marco Longoni, and Elio Agostoni

Abstract All patients with stroke or suspected stroke benefit from integrated stroke care systems which are created following the recommendations in the guidelines of the American Heart Association (AHA)/American Stroke Association (ASA) [1]. These care systems include hospitals for treating acute stroke, which often offer telemedicine and teleradiology, comprehensive stroke units, emergency units, public agencies and government resources. The objectives are prevention of stroke, optimal use of emergency departments, treatment of acute and subacute stroke, rehabilitation and follow-up, as well as educational programmes. Randomized clinical trials have shown that patients treated in primary stroke centres have a better outcome than patients treated in facilities without a stroke unit and that the rate of thrombolysis is higher; thus in the AHA/ASA guidelines, the creation of primary stroke centres is recommended (Class I, Evidence

G. D'Aliberti et al., *Ischemic Stroke*, Emergency Management   87
in Neurology, DOI 10.1007/978-3-319-31705-2_4,
© Springer International Publishing Switzerland 2017

TABLE 4.1 Decisional algorithm

Setting A	
Hospital with:	Emergency department
	24/7 radiology services
	24/7 laboratory services
Setting B	
Hospital with:	Emergency department
	24/7 radiology services
	24/7 laboratory services
	24/7 neurology/stroke unit + hospital neurologist available
Setting C	
Hospital with:	Emergency department
	24/7 radiology services
	24/7 laboratory services
	24/7 neurology/stroke unit
	Neuroradiology/interventional radiology
	Neurosurgery

Level B), pointing out that these centres must be certified by an external organization. They further recommend setting up a multidisciplinary "improvement and quality" commission for reviewing and monitoring quality indicators, such as quality of care, evidence-based practice and prognosis (Class I, Level of Evidence B), in order to identify any deficiencies and to arrange to have them corrected. This chapter presents some algorithms for decision making, inspired not only by the clinical aspects but also by the organizational, technological, and professional characteristics of the hospital receiving and caring for the acute stroke patients. A summarizing table (*decisional algorithm*, Table 4.1) classifies the various settings

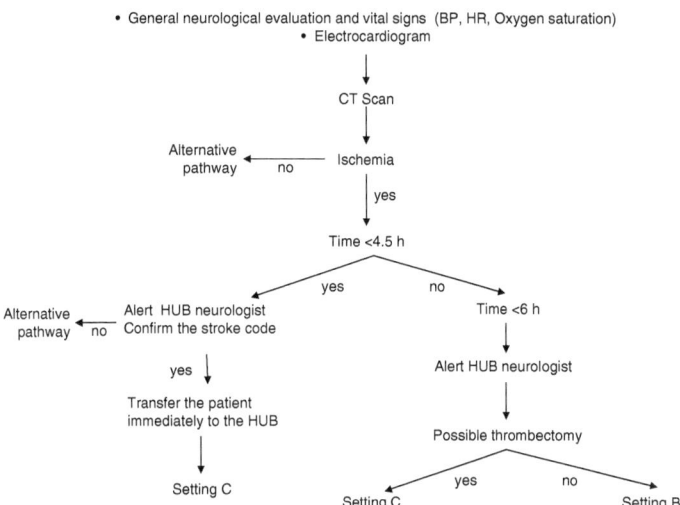

FIGURE 4.1 Setting A. Patients with suspected acute stroke

(A, B, C) in which clinicians manage patients. These algorithms are to be considered as reference material for helping physicians in selecting the most adequate pathway according to the hospital facilities available.

The decisional algorithms are organized and diversified into three main situations (Figs. 4.1, 4.2, and 4.3) that suggest the same number of different practical behaviors aiming at guaranteeing the best care, albeit in different organizational situations. This really brings to the fore the concept of network and of organization through the HUB and Spoke model.

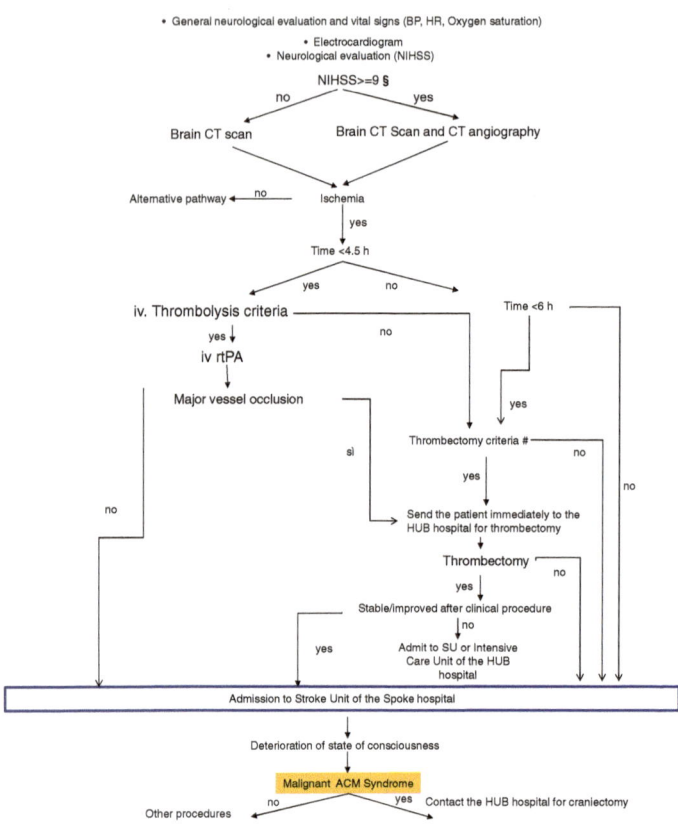

- General neurological evaluation and vital signs (BP, HR, Oxygen saturation)
- Electrocardiogram
- Neurological evaluation (NIHSS)

NIHSS>=9 §

no ← → yes

Brain CT scan   Brain CT Scan and CT angiography

Alternative pathway ← no ── Ischemia

yes

Time <4.5 h

yes ← → no

iv. Thrombolysis criteria ──────   Time <6 h

yes ↓   no

iv rtPA

Major vessel occlusion ──────

no   yes

Thrombectomy criteria #

si   no

yes

no   no

Send the patient immediately to the
HUB hospital for thrombectomy

Thrombectomy   no

yes ↓

Stable/improved after clinical procedure

yes ↓ no

Admit to SU or Intensive
Care Unit of the HUB
hospital

Admission to Stroke Unit of the Spoke hospital

Deterioration of state of consciousness

Malignant ACM Syndrome

no   yes   Contact the HUB hospital for craniectomy

Other procedures

§ for NIHSS values under 9, the CT angiography is carried out according to neurologists' recommendations
# thrombectomy is indicated where there is an occlusion of the carotid arteries, medium cerebral arteries (M1–M2),
anterior cerebral artery (A1), posterior cerebral artery (P1) and basal arteries. The following are considered
selection criteria: Aspect score on the CT scan >6, age below 80 years and presence of collateral circulations.

FIGURE 4.2 Setting B. Patient with suspected acute stroke

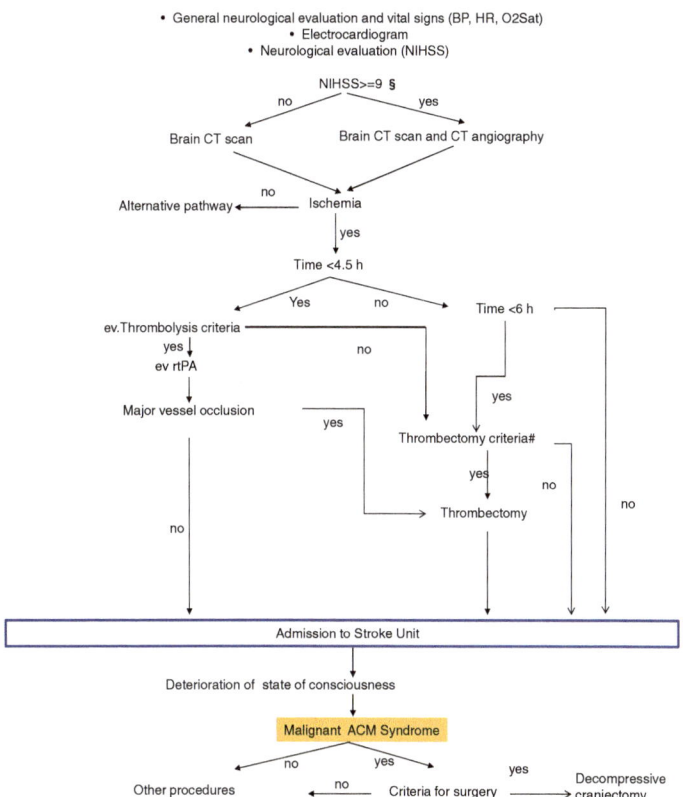

- General neurological evaluation and vital signs (BP, HR, O2Sat)
- Electrocardiogram
- Neurological evaluation (NIHSS)

NIHSS>=9 §

no ← → yes

Brain CT scan | Brain CT scan and CT angiography

no

Alternative pathway ← Ischemia

yes

Time <4.5 h

Yes | no → Time <6 h

ev.Thrombolysis criteria

yes ↓ no

ev rtPA

Major vessel occlusion | yes

yes

Thrombectomy criteria#

yes | no

no

no

Thrombectomy

no

Admission to Stroke Unit

Deterioration of state of consciousness

Malignant ACM Syndrome

no ← → yes

yes

Other procedures | no ← Criteria for surgery → Decompressive craniectomy

§ for NIHSS values under 9, the CT angiography is carried out according to neurologists' recommendations
# thrombectomy is indicated where there is an occlusion of the carotid arteries, medium cerebral arteries (M1–M2). ,anterior cerebral artery (A1), posterior cerebral artery (P1) and basal arteries. The following are considered selection criteria: Aspect score on the CT scan >6, age below 80 years and presence of collateral circulations.

FIGURE 4.3 Setting C. HUB – Patient with suspected acute stroke